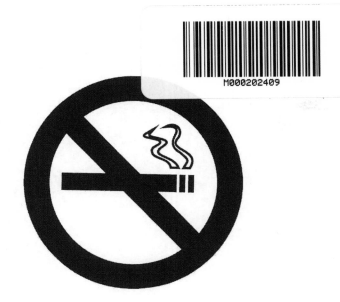

For Smokers Only
How Smokeless Tobacco Can Save Your Life

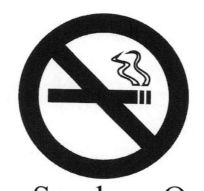

For Smokers Only
How Smokeless Tobacco Can Save Your Life

Brad Rodu, D.D.S.

Professor of Medicine
Endowed Chair, Tobacco Harm Reduction Research
University of Louisville

Sumner Books
Hermosa Beach, CA

For Smokers Only
How Smokeless Tobacco Can Save Your Life
Copyright © 1995, 2014, 2016 Sumner Books

Illustrations: Robin Culver, Sam Miller
Photographs: Rick Daniel

Sumner Books
737 3rd St
Hermosa Beach, California 90254
310-337-7003
ISBN 978-1-939104-30-4
CREATORS PUBLISHING

Dr. Rodu examines and comments on scientific issues surrounding tobacco policies – and fallacies – at his blog: http://rodutobaccotruth.blogspot.com/.

~ ~ ~

Contents

Acknowledgments

During the development of this quit-smoking strategy and its evolution into a book, many colleagues and friends have provided valuable support and guidance. These people came from many personal and professional backgrounds, and each contributed in a special way to this effort. But many of the individuals mentioned below have one thing in common: an ability to look at a new and provocative idea with an open mind, and judge it on its merits. That trait is less common than you might think.

John Masefield, Poet Laureate of England in 1946, described a university as "a place where those who hate ignorance may strive to know; where those who perceive truth may strive to make others see; where seekers and learners alike, banded together in the search for knowledge, will honor thought in all its finer ways." Three faculty members in particular at the University of Alabama at Birmingham have embraced those lofty ideals throughout their careers, and deserve special mention in this section. Ms. Caren Barnes, Professor of Dentistry, served as a valuable resource at key decision-making points in this program over the past few years. Dr. Don Miller, Professor of Medicine and Director of Hematology-Oncology provided insights into critical medical issues with impeccable and almost uncanny timing. And he has done so countless times since our careers crossed a decade ago. Dr. Philip Cole, Professor of Epidemiology, has served as a collaborator on projects related to this idea for the past two years. In this short period he has challenged me to write — even more fundamentally to think — with precision, clarity and refinement about many important facets of the tobacco issue.

The Department of Oral Pathology is a small but productive and efficient medical center unit. It is productive because of fellow oral pathologists Dr. Ken Tilashalski and Dr. Nadarajah Vigneswaran. They have devoted much time and effort into some of the clinical research projects I have cited in this book. The department is efficient because of the administrative and technical support provided by Karen Christian, Karen Rotenberry, and Roger James.

In some respects my colleagues at UAB were fortunate, having to endure the smokeless tobacco idea for only eight hours a day, five days a week. On nights and weekends, my long-suffering family assumed the inevitable duty. I hope the completion of this book serves as modest recompense to Portia, Alexandra and Jordan for involuntarily serving as the sounding board for the lessons and lectures, the plans and programs that surrounded the development of the smokeless tobacco solution. My extended family — consisting essentially of my mother and my brother — also deserve awards for their patience.

This book benefits immensely from a trio of talented artists. Rick Daniel produced the fine photographs which demonstrate with remarkable clarity how easy the smokeless tobacco solution can be. I am also grateful for the assistance of two students at the University of Alabama, Robin Culver and Sam Miller. Their artwork powerfully portrays the despair facing so many cigarette smokers and the hope that the smokeless tobacco solution offers them.

March 2014
Special Acknowledgments

I want to take this opportunity to acknowledge the unfailing support of my efforts for over 20 years by Mr. William Sklar.

I met Mr. Sklar in 1987, when I was conducting contract research for a pharmaceutical company as a faculty member at UAB. I immediately recognized that Mr. Sklar was a brilliant and creative writer with broad understanding of and valuable insights into legislative, regulatory and policy perspectives.

When I was writing *For Smokers Only* in 1994, Mr. Sklar agreed to serve as behind-the-scene editor. He developed a comprehensive understanding of the scientific and medical foundation for tobacco harm reduction, and provided a valuable sounding board as I translated complicated medical and epidemiologic concepts into clear public health messages for the nation's 45 million smokers.

Since then, Mr. Sklar has been my editor and advisor for innumerable letters to editors, presentations, commentaries, Congressional testimony and more. In my original Acknowledgment

I recognized other individuals who played important roles in the development of the book, but Mr. Sklar is the only collaborator who was there when the idea was born, and is still offering invaluable guidance and advice today. I am most grateful for his assistance and friendship.

I also want to express special thanks to Rick Newcombe for publishing the electronic version of the book. This acknowledgment is long overdue. In 1998, Mr. Newcombe, who had read *For Smokers Only* and had become a regular correspondent, offered to obtain the copyright and make a fresh print run under the auspices of his publishing company, Sumner Books. With that gesture he kept the "smoke-free" flame alive for over a decade. Earlier this year, Mr. Newcombe offered to publish *For Smokers Only* as an e-book, complete with a new chapter on e-cigarettes. I am thrilled to bring this work into the digital age and to extend my 20-year quest to help smokers enjoy longer and healthier lives.

The e-venture was accomplished with the able assistance of Peter Kaminski, Aimee Kuvadia, Heather Schultz and Brandon Telle at Sumner Books.

John Maguire kindly supplied photographs of smokeless tobacco products and e-cigarettes.

~ ~ ~

About the Author

Dr. Brad Rodu was Chair of Oral Pathology at the University of Alabama at Birmingham when he published *For Smokers Only* in 1995. Since then, he has been in the forefront of research and policy development regarding tobacco harm reduction – permanent nicotine maintenance with safer tobacco products by smokers who are unable or unwilling to quit smoking with conventional cessation methods.

At UAB, Dr. Rodu held positions in several departments in the Schools of Medicine, Public Health and Dentistry. In 2005, he moved to the University of Louisville as Professor of Medicine and was appointed as the first holder of an Endowed Chair in Tobacco Harm Reduction Research at the James Graham Brown Cancer Center.

Dr. Rodu has authored or co-authored 40 peer-reviewed professional publications regarding tobacco that have appeared in a broad range of medical and scientific journals, including *Nature*, *The American Journal of Medicine*, *Epidemiology* and *Journal of Clinical Oncology*. He has written commentaries for the general press and served as an expert witness at a 2003 Congressional hearing on tobacco harm reduction. Dr. Rodu has spoken at international forums, including one at the British Houses of Parliament, and has testified at numerous state legislative hearings.

A native of Ohio, Dr. Rodu earned his dental degree from the Ohio State University in 1977. After an oral pathology residency at Emory University, Dr. Rodu completed fellowships at the University of Alabama at Birmingham that were sponsored by the American Cancer Society and the National Cancer Institute.

Funding Our Research

Every university research project has financial costs for salaries, office space, computers and other necessary resources. When I wrote *For Smokers Only* in 1994, our tobacco harm reduction research was supported solely by department funds. By 1999, I had authored 10 professional articles in peer-reviewed journals, but money was running low. A secure funding source was needed.

The National Institutes of Health should have supported our work, but in 1995 the National Cancer Institute had launched an unjustified attack on our tobacco research and credibility; this was chronicled by Jacob Sullum in his book, *For Your Own Good.* Our only viable alternative was the tobacco industry.

Starting in 1999, our research was funded by unrestricted grants from tobacco manufacturers to the University of Alabama at Birmingham, and then the University of Louisville, where they have been administered according to stringent university policies. The terms of the grants have assured the complete independence of our research and its publication with respect to any influence or interference from sponsors. I live on a university professor's salary, and have no personal conflicts of interest with any stakeholder in tobacco issues.

~ ~ ~

Foreword

This book is for you.

It was written for you, the mature adult smoker who wants to quit. You have tried at least several times to give up smoking. You made the effort on your own, or perhaps with the help of a quit-smoking program. Whatever your approach, it brought little or no success. Now, you are deeply concerned about what your habit is doing to you. It was bad enough when you were concerned only about the effects on your own health. But lately additional worries have emerged over the effects of your smoking on the health of your family. And, to top it all off, you are gradually becoming a social outcast. Many aspects of your life now seem somewhat the worse because you smoke.

Why, then, are you unable to quit? Frankly, the answer is that you are physically, and perhaps psychologically, dependent on the nicotine that smoking provides. Quit-smoking plans that require you to give up nicotine are likely to fail in the future as they have in the past. That is exactly why this book is for you: it recognizes your difficulty and it uniquely provides a new way in which you can give up smoking without tormenting yourself by trying to give up nicotine. Another strong point of this book is that it delivers only a scientifically-based educational message; there is no effort to coerce you or to make you feel guilty. In these ways it is different from other quit-smoking plans and from the efforts of the modern-day prohibitionists who, believe it or not, wish to ban all tobacco products.

The plan put forward in this book is simple and it works. It works because it does not deprive you of the nicotine that your body craves. You may respond to my brief description of this plan with something between curiosity and, perhaps, repugnance. But for your own sake hear me out, because your curiosity can be satisfied and your negative response is probably based on out-of-date views.

The plan is that you will substitute smokeless tobacco for smoking. The underlying reasoning is simple and correct: it is the smoke from a cigarette, not the nicotine, that causes disease. Yet, smokeless tobacco easily provides enough nicotine to satisfy your craving and poses a minimal health risk to you. This risk is estimated to be less than two percent as large as the risk associated with smoking. And as fringe benefits, smokeless tobacco poses no risk to anyone else and its use is sufficiently discreet that you will not be ostracized in any way.

Do you find the idea of using smokeless tobacco repugnant? If so, you may have an outmoded image of "chewing" tobacco: perhaps you envision a somewhat unsavory character with a bulging cheek looking for a spittoon. But a modern smokeless product involves none of this. Instead, this book offers you a socially acceptable, safe way of satisfying your craving for nicotine. Be open-minded. Read the book. Give the plan a try.

I met the author of this book, Dr. Brad Rodu, two years ago. He is an oral pathologist and a researcher. I was at first surprised by what he had to say. Yet my intuition told me from the start that he was on to something. But we cannot rely on intuition for preventing disease: we require facts, hard facts. Dr. Rodu has them and there is simply no controverting the information he has put together. I know because I have tried.

Dr. Rodu's smokeless tobacco plan, "if you can't quit, switch," is based on common sense. In fact, more than one million smokers saw this for themselves and made the switch on their own. Dr. Rodu's special contribution is that he has done thorough research and brought clearthinking to the problem at hand: What to do for the persistent smoker? Dr. Rodu wants you to quit if you can, but he has accepted the reality that many smokers can quit only if they have an alternative. Dr. Rodu also warrants commendation for the courage he has shown in advancing his plan, for he has not yet received the endorsement of the public health community. Eventually the endorsement will be forthcoming because Dr. Rodu's contribution is straightforward. He has assembled the information that establishes the safety and acceptability of modern smokeless tobacco products as a substitute for smoking. He wants you to give this approach a try for no reason but one: you will be much, much better off if you use smokeless tobacco instead of cigarettes. This book documents that statement to be true and shows you how to make the switch.

Philip Cole, M.D., Dr.P.H.
Professor of Epidemiology, UAB

~ ~ ~

7

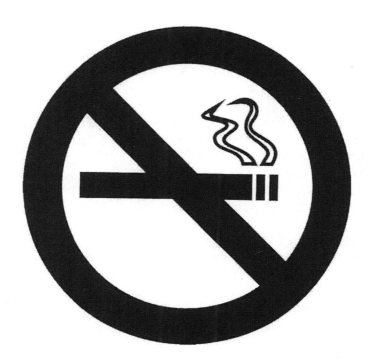

Introduction

Introduction

Tobacco is a dirty weed: I like it.
It satisfies no normal need: I like it.
It makes you thin, it makes you lean,
It takes the hair right off your bean;
It's the worst darn stuff I've ever seen: I like it.

— Graham Hemminger
Tobacco: Penn State Froth
November 1915

What This Book Is About

This book intends to help the 46 million people in the United States who still smoke despite the Surgeon General reports, cancer and lung disease statistics, insurance rate and tax hikes, and the more recent no-smoking bans in public places.

Too many intelligent people continue to smoke. Obviously, these smokers are hooked by a physical addiction that speaks louder than common sense. This controversial book, therefore, will do more than provide informational and motivational facts to move smokers away from cigarettes. It will offer them a physically and logically viable alternative to cigarettes in the form of smokeless tobacco products.

Now, put all your prejudices and misconceptions on hold and give this book a fair chance. If you or your loved one is a cigarette smoker, you cannot afford to ignore the facts, arguments, and workable solutions offered here.

This is a no-nonsense guide to the facts and fallacies of various kinds of tobacco use. This is the first book by a health professional that speaks to the smoker with sympathy and practicality, and that offers the smoker real choices.

Today health professionals essentially give you only an ultimatum: Quit smoking or suffer the consequences. Their only option to smoking — total tobacco abstinence — is one that many smokers cannot or will not choose, especially in time to prevent the many dire health problems associated with the habit.

You may have been badgered and lectured by your doctor to quit smoking. Let me give you some advice: Don't just pay attention to your doctor's warnings; pay more attention to your doctor's actions.

Chances are he or she has never started smoking or has quit. Recent surveys show that less than ten percent of doctors now smoke cigarettes. They are in the know. They have read hundreds of journals, research papers, and autopsy reports. Don't let smoke get in your eyes. If you can't buck the craving, be flexible enough to get alternative tobacco satisfaction that won't get your name on your doctor's upcoming autopsy report.

Because of your physical and psychological need for cigarettes, smokeless tobacco presents you with an imperfect but entirely viable solution. I will discuss the various smokeless tobacco products, what's in them, how they are used, and the health implications in later chapters. For now, let me say that smokeless tobacco products allow you, the hard-core and long-term smoker, to take back a measure of control over your health by indulging in a far safer form of tobacco use. This book provides accurate information and easy-to-follow instructions that will change your life for the better.

You have every right to be skeptical about my thesis. The media has inundated you with indiscriminate attacks against tobacco and nicotine by way of condemning cigarettes. (Throwing out the baby with the bath water seems to be a national sport in the 1990's.) While I do not advocate tobacco use of any kind, you will be pleasantly surprised to learn that tobacco and nicotine themselves are not the major problems. By the time you finish this book, you will see that I am not merely indulging you with an easy, lesser-of-two-evils solution, and I am not cynically suggesting that you trade lung cancer for oral cancer. This issue is far more important. With this information, I am offering you the opportunity to enjoy a healthier and longer life.

What This Book Is Not About

There are a couple of things that this book is not. First, it is not a blanket endorsement of any kind of tobacco product. It is very clear that use of tobacco in any manner is a health-risky venture. In an ideal world, it would be preferable for you to give up tobacco altogether. For this reason, I am including material on other programs for quitting smoking. I do point out weaknesses in these smoke-ending programs, but anything that might work is commendable. Studies show, however, that most people who quit smoking do so on their own, without the assistance of expensive and time-consuming products or therapists.

A visit to a large bookstore reveals an almost empty "How-To" shelf with regard to quitting smoking. The thinking American smoker is left with faddish and incomplete magazine articles on the topic. You deserve more. In layman's language, I want to go broadly and deeply on the topic of tobacco to reach your heart and mind — and your lungs, too.

This is also not a book on tobacco initiation. How people come to be cigarette smokers is a complex and difficult subject. It is clear that many smokers started when they were teenagers, when they had little or no regard for the future health implications of a lifetime of cigarette consumption. Critics may argue that this book will encourage teenagers to pick up the smokeless tobacco habit. But anyone reading the entire book will learn that, by detailing all of the health risks associated with tobacco use, introducing nonsmokers to smokeless tobacco is the furthest thing from my intentions.

Before branding me as that reckless doctor who recommends exchanging spittoons for ashtrays, take a moment to carefully consider the limitations of my thesis. As you will read in the forthcoming chapters, I strongly recommend that everyone refrain from all nicotine and tobacco products. Smokeless tobacco is only suggested as a realistic, immediate, and permanent solution for the addicted smoker.

The nation's 46 million smokers need help to loosen the shackles of the smoking habit. And let's face it, if they haven't quit smoking by now, the odds — and the clock — are working against them. These smokers need a workable solution that is going to meet their physical needs, while reducing a plethora of deadly dangers to themselves and others. This book, as well as the smokeless tobacco solution, is for them.

I want this controversial book to be thoroughly unnecessary within a generation. Smokeless tobacco should only provide a viable and comparatively safe damage control measure for the current and last generation of nicotine addicts. Forty years or so from now I hope there are no tobacco users left on the planet. But hope alone will not prevent the 419,000 smoking-related deaths that will occur in the United States this year (that's 1,150 fatalities every day). Smokeless tobacco may provide a stay of execution for some of the 46 million American smokers on this seemingly endless death-row list.

By providing an alternative nicotine delivery system, the smokeless tobacco solution has been compared to providing methadone to heroin addicts. If you think methadone and heroin addiction are too harsh for metaphors in a book about tobacco, then you are underestimating the power of nicotine addiction and ignoring the fact that cigarettes kill thousands more a year than hypodermic needles full of "junk."

The Methadone-Smokeless Tobacco Analogy

Comparing my thesis to the now widespread and successful treatment of heroin addicts with methadone is more apt than you think. I expect the same kind of resistance and harsh criticism from the unimaginative medical establishment that the proponents of methadone substitution received years ago. Examination of this issue reveals important lessons regarding the relationship between scientific and medical facts and resulting public health policy.

In 1964, addiction experts Vincent Dole and Marie Nyswander responded to the dangerous increase in shooting-up heroin by testing an oral drug, methadone, that could safely substitute for the junk the addicts craved. Three years after publishing the results of their work in the Journal of the American Medical Association in 1965, they were successfully treating 1,100 former addicts. Within ten years over 80,000 former heroin addicts were helped in their methadone maintenance treatment (MMT).

Do you think the medical community welcomed their innovative idea with open arms? No. There was a deafening roar of disapproval, or what was described as "a heated debate during which clinical experience and the derived scientific data were ignored." The real fight was about "philosophical differences — objections to the substitution of one drug for another" rather than doubts about the safety and effectiveness of the methadone treatments. Public debates about addictions like nicotine or heroin (but not caffeine, as I'll discuss in Chapter Five) focus on intensely subjective and philosophical issues, and the resulting public health policies are shaped more by emotion and intuition than by scientific evidence.

This situation has eerie parallels to our tobacco problem. Instead of concern for the lives of cigarette junkies, some purists are fighting the concept of trading in one form of tobacco for another. Addictive drugs like heroin and nicotine cannot be wished away. When junkies are shooting up, killing themselves and others, one is grateful for a safer alternative. When smokers are killing themselves and placing the people around them at risk, one should also look for a safer tobacco substitute.

In both situations, the alternative oral delivery systems (methadone and smokeless tobacco) are much safer than the hypodermic needle or the paper tube of inhaled chemical fumes. The analogy here is instructive, but not airtight. Heroin is illegal and its users cannot lead productive lives. In addition, methadone does involve the substitution of one drug for another. At least for now, tobacco products are legal, and my solution to your smoking predicament involves the same drug you are already using — nicotine. There are other nicotine delivery systems, like the nicotine patch or gum (see Chapter Six), that can serve as alternatives to cigarettes, and I am all for them. But these prescription products have failed for many smokers. Since smokeless tobacco is acceptable to the smoker and is inexpensive, available and satisfying, it is the MMT program that can realistically combat smoking.

Admittedly, this safer form of tobacco might become too attractive, to the point of creating some new addicts. I would therefore like widespread health education against smoking and all tobacco use to specifically target teenagers, too many of whom are developing nicotine addictions through cigarettes or smokeless tobacco. My proposal to switch to snuff is only a second-best measure for addicted veteran smokers who cannot quit. I do *not* advocate nonsmokers taking up smokeless tobacco as a "safe" or "safer" habit. While I have compassion for older smokers who feel they need a regular fix to work or relax properly, no legislation limiting youth access to tobacco can be tough enough.

Just What is Smokeless Tobacco?

There are many people in the nation's big cities who are not quite sure what smokeless tobacco is. Yes, it includes the wads or plugs of loose leaf tobacco bulging in the cheeks of baseball players and coaches. That is called chewing tobacco, and it involves some manly, but ungentlemanly (and not at all ladylike), spitting of saliva and tobacco juices. In this text the recommended switch for most

13

smokers will be what is called moist snuff. "Dippers" of moist snuff place a pinch or a tiny pouch of tobacco between their cheek and gum. It is more discreet than chewing gum, and it is as easy to use as a breath mint. The health officials who like to call snuff "spit tobacco" have it wrong: there is little or no excess saliva involved.

While the neater, spitless forms of smokeless tobacco have become more popular in recent years, especially with women, it is the burning of cigarettes that turned tobacco use into the deadly menace it is today. Back in 1900, 60 percent of the seven and one-half pounds of tobacco consumed per adult in the United States was smokeless. More on the history and how-to's of smokeless tobacco will be discussed later in the text, but this brief note was necessary here for those cigarette smokers who never imagined that a smokeless tobacco product could be enjoyed off the baseball diamond or farmhouse porch.

Those baseball players, with cheeks full of tobacco and long streams of spit, are admittedly poor representatives of the finer art of enjoying smokeless products. The comical close-ups of these puff-cheeked spitters are increasingly rare because the vast majority of the 37 percent of ballplayers who use smokeless tobacco now use snuff. Most importantly, the 46 million smokers facing serious diseases cannot laugh at these ballplayers. Only 3 percent of ballplayers smoke, and a whopping 88 percent of them have never smoked (percentages very similar to those I reported earlier for physicians). Instead of condemning ballplayers as a bunch of unhealthy tobacco users, one should note how few of them come down with all the cancers, heart, and respiratory ailments of the smoking population.

My final introductory word is "enjoy." Smokers tend to have a strong streak of hedonism along with a well-developed sense of denial. This book will make denial of smoking's dangers impossible, but it does not deny the smoker's pursuit of pleasure. You can have your tobacco and enjoy it too.

~ ~ ~

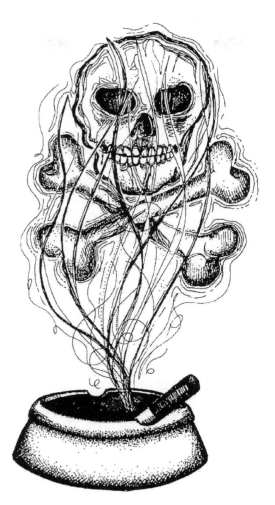

Chapter One
Common Questions and Uncommon Answers

Chapter One
Common Questions and Uncommon Answers

For thy sake, Tobacco,
I would do anything but die.

— Charles Lamb
(1775-1834)

My program to help cigarette smokers make the switch to smokeless tobacco has raised a lot of eyebrows, and people have asked a lot of questions. The most common questions and their condensed answers here will give you a preview of the major issues. Myths and misconceptions die hard, so feel free to follow up the brief responses here with comprehensive discussions in later chapters.

Q. *Why are you suggesting that smokers take up another form of tobacco when they need to quit nicotine altogether?*

A. There is no doubt that all tobacco users should do just what you say — quit nicotine completely. But that is the ideal, and we live in a real world. We know that nicotine causes a powerful addiction that many people just cannot shake. Neither life-threatening situations (see Chapter Three) nor smoke-quitting devices and programs (see Chapter Six) have been successful in helping enough smokers quit.

Read Chapter Five for a description of the symptoms of nicotine addiction. In fact, nicotine addiction is powerful enough and cigarette smoking is dangerous enough to compare my smokeless tobacco alternative to the methadone treatment given to heroin junkies (see the Introduction). Methadone, like snuff or plug tobacco, is no cure, but it is a way to keep the junkie from killing himself or others with his need for heroin.

The cigarette smoker is clearly killing himself (see Chapter Three) and possibly those around him (see Chapter Four) with the deadly fumes of his nicotine delivery system. A switch to a safer delivery system, smokeless tobacco, will allow the 46 million smokers in this country (and the people they live with) to live longer, healthier lives. That is the realistic and compelling message of this book that needs to be shouted from the mountain tops.

Q. *Aren't the figures on deaths caused by smoking and on the billions of dollars that smoking costs us in health care just a lot of hype from antitobacco activists?*

A. Not really. The statistics on deaths from smoking-related heart and lung diseases and cancers (see Chapter Three) are quite sound and very frightening. Smoking is the greatest identifiable and preventable cause of premature deaths. The anti-tobacco lobby is guilty of exaggeration when it comes to pinning our national health care crisis on smokers, but the cigarette industry cannot escape the fact that the smoker who literally dies for a cigarette loses up to fifteen years of life. The widows and widowers left behind for all those lonely years will not be comforted by arguments about health care costs and increasing tobacco taxes.

My lifesaving program may be irrationally dismissed because I haven't declared all tobacco and nicotine products to be the devil's tools (see Chapter Eight). Caffeine is also an addictive substance that can be abused, but it is enjoyed relatively safely and therefore is not a target in the general crusade against drug addiction. In fact, caffeine and nicotine are remarkably similar; I think you'll be surprised by my comparison in Chapter Five.

Q. *I read that many smokeless tobacco products have just as much nicotine in them as cigarettes, so all you accomplish by switching from cigarettes to snuff is killing yourself without harming others with your secondhand smoke. Aren't you advocating an alternative form of suicide by recommending smokeless tobacco?*

A. You are right that smokeless tobacco products can have the same amount of nicotine — or more — than various brands of cigarettes (see Chapter Seven). That's exactly what makes snuff satisfying enough to allow smokers to quit puffing on those coffin nails. The many noxious chemicals in tobacco smoke, not in tobacco or nicotine itself, are the major killers (see Chapter Five). Far from an alternative suicide, my plan offers smokers many more years of health and life (see Chapter Seven). But remember that as good as the smokeless tobacco solution is, the only way to avoid tobacco risks entirely is to avoid tobacco entirely.

Q. *Can't they make the right kind of filter or low tar cigarette that can be safer to smoke?*

A. The cigarette companies have spent a lot of time and money trying to make this seemingly logical but practically impossible idea a reality. Filters only make smokers pay more for less tobacco and force them to puff harder and more often to get the same amount of nicotine their bodies need. As long as smokers inhale the combustion products of tobacco, the risk for cancers, lung diseases, and heart problems remain high. See Chapter Five for why the harmful by-products of smoking may have nothing to do with filters or tar content.

Q. *I read that smokeless tobacco gives you oral cancer. Why would you advocate switching from lung cancer to mouth cancer?*

A. Switching from lung cancer to mouth cancer is an inaccurate oversimplification. In Chapter Seven you will see that users of snuff are only slightly more at risk for mouth cancer than nonsmokers. The kinds of mouth cancers that can develop from smokeless tobacco use are quite detectable and treatable, especially when compared to the many cancers clearly associated with cigarette smoking. Throughout this book I will never claim smokeless tobacco to be a perfect, hazard-free alternative to smoking. It is only a godsend when compared to the plethora of deadly toxins that smokers pour into their system.

Q. *I tried the nicotine patch and the nicotine gum. Nothing kept me from relapsing months after having "quit for good." What makes you think that smokeless tobacco will be any more effective in helping me quit smoking completely?*

A. I know what you are going through, because many former smokers crave nicotine for the rest of their lives. The nicotine gum and patch neutralized your nicotine addiction in the short run, but didn't offer you the tobacco pleasure your body and mind craved (see Chapter Six). One fundamental dilemma of programs employing prescription nicotine substitution is that they eventually require you to quit nicotine entirely, a proposition which your body may continuously rebel against. With smokeless tobacco you can enjoy full-bodied tobacco flavor (and nicotine), and I am confident that you will find the right product that will make you forget how to light a match.

Q. *I gained almost fifteen pounds when I quit smoking for a while. I would try your idea, but I just can't let myself balloon up like that again. What do you suggest?*

A. The weight gain associated with quitting smoking is an added reason why so many stop-smoking programs end up in failure. Longtime nicotine use is a major part of smoking that has affected your metabolism and appetite (see Chapter Six). When you quit, your nicotine withdrawal and craving is accompanied by hassles in maintaining the weight and metabolic rate that you became comfortable with when smoking. You can do that easily with smokeless tobacco. But if you don't give up cigarettes immediately, you may be one more trim looking smoker whose life is tragically and avoidably cut short.

Q. *I understand and appreciate all you said about switching to smokeless. But I'm a lady, not a ballplayer. Do you expect me to stand there and spit tobacco juice like a shortstop?*

A. Of course not. What you should try are those tiny, discreet pouches of snuff that are as undetectable as a breath mint. Very little or no excess saliva is produced. (The easy mechanics for this switch in Chapter Seven are for women too.) You will no longer look like a classy lady who spews out noxious smoke and ash.

You are probably thinking of the baseball players and rodeo riders with big wads of chewing tobacco bulging in their cheeks. A lot less macho and much more ladylike are the small packets of snuff that allow you to enjoy tobacco discreetly and with the best of etiquette. As women jogging on the sidewalk was outrageous in 1958 but normal today, so it should be socially acceptable for a woman today to use smokeless tobacco "or medicinal purposes." Your "lifetime" batting average against cancer and lung and heart disease will also be far better.

Q. *If I swallow some of the juices from chewing tobacco won't I get sick, maybe with cancer of the stomach or colon?*

A. Swallowing tobacco juice may upset your stomach, but researchers have never been able to link stomach or other cancers to long-term smokeless tobacco use — despite years of searching. Any swallowing or spitting of tobacco juice is at a minimum with today's smokeless tobacco products and is not a problem for most switchers.

Q. *How am I going to get the nicotine I need without smoking? Do I have to swallow the tobacco or juice to get satisfaction?*

A. Nicotine is efficiently absorbed in the system through the lining of the cheek. Inhaling is, thankfully, irrelevant here, and swallowing does no good because nicotine is poorly absorbed once it hits the acidic conditions in the stomach (see Chapter Five).

Q. *Where do I place the smokeless tobacco? How long do I keep it there? How often should I use it each day?*

A. The small pouch of snuff or pinch of tobacco is placed between the cheek and gum. Some users are satisfied after ten minutes, while others like to nurse their dip for an hour or more. Each application not only lasts longer than a cigarette, but the nicotine stays in your bloodstream longer. A thirty-cigarette-a-day smoker will probably not need more than a few pouches of snuff a day, but each individual's tastes and needs will dictate use. See Chapter Seven for a more detailed look at how to use smokeless tobacco.

Q. *Can I still smoke cigarettes but use smokeless tobacco to reduce the number that I smoke?*

A. It is possible to use this program to cut down gradually on smoking, but I don't recommend it. First, unlike other quitting strategies, you never have to go cold turkey. The smokeless tobacco is your smoking substitute, providing the nicotine your body craves. Second, smokers who simply cut back a bit may be kidding themselves. At least for lung cancer, studies have shown that risks may remain high for the few cigarettes-a-day smoker because of the daily bombardment by the cancer-causing chemicals in smoke. Check out the good news in Chapter Six on when you quit for keeps.

Q. *What can I do to use smokeless tobacco invisibly? I often find myself in delicate social situations.*

A. You should stick with the neat little packets of moist snuff, beginning with the variety of flavors and strengths offered by brands like Skoal Bandits. Read the charts in Chapter Seven to help you experiment with a brand that you can enjoy. There is no visible sign that you are enjoying tobacco when this little paper pouch is nestled comfortably between your cheek and gum.

After a few days, you'll feel comfortable enough with the pouch to keep one in your mouth during a high pressure business presentation or while hosting a gala social event. These nervous times are precisely when you reach for your pack of cigarettes. That same calming effect that helps you work better when you smoke will be available to you with smokeless tobacco. In addition, you will be avoiding the intense (and possibly even unfair) criticism resulting from the secondhand smoke debate (see Chapter Four).

Q. *I don't have to stop smoking because there is no lung cancer in my family. There is some history of heart disease, but eating right and dieting will keep me healthy. And isn't it true that smoking can't be strongly linked to strokes and heart attacks?*

A. You are playing a dangerous game with a little bit of medical information. There are cancers of the larynx, esophagus, and elsewhere that smokers have to worry about, not merely lung cancer (see Chapter Three). Diet and exercise do not reverse a budding heart problem, and a disproportionate number of smokers do die prematurely of strokes and heart attacks. Don't think smoking doesn't cause heart disease just because researchers can't tell you which chemical in smoke is the culprit.

To the statisticians who count death certificates, the exact cause isn't relevant. What is relevant is that your name is not on one of those certificates prematurely.

Q. *What will my family physician or dentist say when I tell him about my decision to try smokeless tobacco?*

A. If your physician has any integrity and depth, she or he will not judge smokeless tobacco by the medical establishment's knee-jerk condemnation (see Chapter Eight). Doctors are noted for their independence, and they will not let the nation's medical organizations cloud their own analysis of my research. Why not lend your doctors a copy of this book to help them form an opinion? If your doctors do not applaud your giving up smoking, then something is very wrong. Don't worry about sounding like a fool; your lungs are going to sound a lot better in a matter of weeks.

You should tell your dentist about your new use of smokeless tobacco. Get regular checkups for gum problems and small white patches of wrinkled skin in the mouth called leukoplakia (see Chapter Seven).

Q. *Will my family and friends make fun of me for using smokeless tobacco?*

A. It is possible, though they might never know if you kept a tiny little bag of snuff in your cheek. The point of the switch to smokeless is to be around long enough for your friends to get used to you. If they would rather see you puffing and wheezing than dipping then it's time to keep the smokeless tobacco and spit out the friends.

Q. *Will my teenagers want to try smokeless tobacco when they see me using it?*

A. Definitely. Smokeless tobacco is already too popular among teens, especially when the goal is for it to be used only by the last generation of nicotine addicted smokers. Explain to your teenager that nicotine addiction has enslaved you for life, and that the smokeless tobacco you use is only the equivalent of a heroin junkie taking methadone treatments. It would be a better idea to take the more discreet pouches of snuff that cannot be detected. At least you are no longer encouraging your teen to smoke and no longer impairing his or her health with secondhand smoke.

Q. *I am wearing a partial denture/dental implant/bridge. Will smokeless tobacco affect the dental work?*

A. There may be some staining, which can be cleaned with ease, but no harm to the dental work. But you should be very familiar with this, because nothing stains dental work more than smoking.

Q. *After I use smokeless tobacco for a while, what changes should I look for in my mouth?*

A. Let your dentist look twice a year for some of the possible effects of longtime smokeless tobacco use, such as gum changes and white areas (see Chapter Seven).

Q. *Is spitting really necessary? And how much will I have to spit?*

A. Many successful switchers in my program don't find it necessary to spit. Others choose to, but because the pouches are small, the amount is minimal and easy to hide (see Chapter Seven).

Q. *Is there any difference between the various brands of smokeless tobacco?*

A. There is a big difference. Plug tobacco, loose leaf chewing tobacco, dry snuff, moist snuff and pouches are all used differently, and there are multiple brand names for every type. Follow my advice in Chapter Seven for sorting through all the choices at your local store.

Q. *When I was a teenager, I tried some chewing tobacco and I felt pretty sick. I'm a fairly heavy smoker now, but why should I try something again that I didn't like the first time?*

A. If you are a smoker who can't quit, you should try some form of smokeless tobacco as a matter of life and breath. You probably didn't build up a tolerance for any tobacco products when you were that young, and your first cigarettes likely made you as dizzy and nauseous as your first chew. Follow my advice in Chapter Seven and start off with a snuff product that best matches your current smoking pattern.

Q. *I've been smoking menthol cigarettes. Which brand of smokeless tobacco should I use?*

A. A menthol smoker should feel right at home with brands of moist snuff such as Skoal Bandits mint or wintergreen flavors. Hawken has a lower nicotine level, while Skoal regular and long cut varieties of Wintergreen are higher in nicotine (see Chapter Seven).

Q. *How much does smokeless tobacco cost? How does the cost differ from cigarettes?*

A. No matter how you cut it, smokeless tobacco is far more economical. You get more tobacco flavor and nicotine kick from the snuff or chewing tobacco on a pound-for-pound basis. Because the nicotine stays in your bloodstream longer with smokeless tobacco, several pouches of snuff can often take the place of an entire pack of cigarettes (see Chapters Five and Seven).

The monetary price you pay for cigarettes is only the start. You should also be worried about the medical ills and bills (see Chapter Three). This is where smokeless tobacco will really save you.

Q. *If smokeless tobacco is just nicotine substitution, why don't the prescription smoke-quitting products work?*

A. Prescription nicotine substitutes, including the patch and gum discussed in Chapter Six, do work for some smokers. But these products fail to help many others because they do not provide blood nicotine levels which prevent craving and withdrawal.

Q. *Can I use smokeless tobacco where smoking is prohibited?*

A. It has become increasingly difficult to find public places where smoking is permitted (see Chapter Four), but none of the new, strict laws cover all forms of tobacco use. Only cigarette smoking is prohibited, extinguishing the perilous secondhand smoke.

Q. *I've been told by my doctor that I have a heart problem. How will smokeless tobacco affect it?*

A. I don't recommend tobacco for anyone, especially someone with a heart problem. However, the fastest way to lower your risk for a serious cardiovascular catastrophe is to stop smoking now (see Chapter Six), and smokeless tobacco can help you do it.

Q. *What if smokeless tobacco doesn't satisfy my craving for a cigarette?*

A. I can understand if you are referring to the familiar rituals of tapping, lighting, flicking, puffing, and stubbing out cigarettes. You fear that your fingers will be free enough to get bored after a switch to smokeless. After some time you may develop your own rituals of using snuff, but I seriously doubt you will have cravings for deep tobacco flavor and that nicotine feeling unless you have chosen a brand of smokeless that is too weak for your tastes. Within the range of smokeless tobacco products, you will find a flavor and potency that equals your cigarette smoking patterns (see Chapter Seven).

Q. *I am already 60 years old and have smoked for 35 years. How will this benefit me?*

A. It's definitely true that the sooner a smoker quits, the greater the potential benefits. Nonetheless, the health benefits of your quitting now are profound, regardless of your age (see Chapter Six).

Q. *What about the warnings on smokeless tobacco products? They mention gum disease, tooth loss, and mouth cancer and say that "this product is not a safe alternative to cigarettes?"*

A. Not even potato chips or nature hikes are "safe." If we look at "safe" to mean relatively safe or "safer," something the government warnings inanely avoid here, then use of smokeless tobacco products is far safer than cigarette smoking. This book is an invitation only for smokers to switch, not a blind endorsement of any tobacco product.

Chapter Seven will spell out how much safer snuff is than cigarettes, to the tune of thousands of lives saved a year. Statistical dangers of using smokeless tobacco do exist, but they are considerably smaller than the dangers related to smoking cigarettes. Gum and tooth problems do not automatically follow smokeless tobacco use; they are a better bet among regular candy eaters who never brush. Twice yearly checkups will monitor and treat any possible problem resulting from the long-term use of snuff. After you read Chapter Seven, you'll look at the warnings on smokeless tobacco products from a different perspective.

Q. *If smokeless tobacco is a safer alternative to cigarette smoking, why isn't it advertised by the smokeless tobacco companies?*

A. In the context of a solution for the smoker who can't quit, it should but never will be advertised. The smokeless tobacco companies are part of the industry and cannot afford to anger their big brothers by admitting that even filter tip and "low tar and nicotine" brands are deadly killers. Furthermore, there are lots of governmental restrictions for advertising smokeless tobacco products. The message about the life-and-death importance of switching has to instead come from a more honest, independent, and courageous medical profession (see Chapter Eight).

Q. *The research behind your switch-to-smokeless idea looks solid. But aren't you just a shill for the smokeless tobacco industry?*

A. Not a chance. This issue is just too important. First, the cigarette makers can't be happy with all the research I quote which indicts cigarettes as major killers. Second, I don't go easy on smokeless tobacco either. I want smokers who can't quit to switch to smokeless tobacco in order to save their lives — not to save the tobacco industry. I hope that all tobacco products can be phased out entirely in a generation. My motivation? This program makes great medical and practical sense. It has helped many former smokers. It can help you.

~ ~ ~

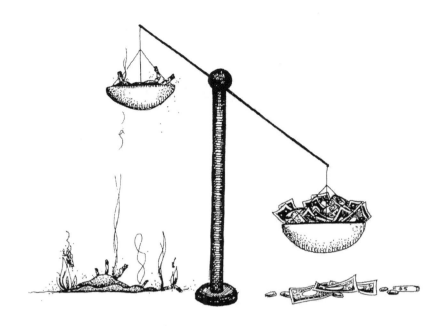

Chapter Two
Getting Up to Snuff: A Brief Tobacco History

Chapter Two
Getting Up to Snuff: A Brief Tobacco History

Chewing tobacco is today's body,
smoke is its ghost, and snuff is tobacco's soul.

— B. C. Stevens
The Collector's Book of Snuff Bottles
(New York, John Weatherhill Inc., 1976)

History's Long Tobacco Road

Anthropologists and historians are sure that tobacco has been used by humans for at least a thousand years. The plant is a New World native and was completely unknown outside the Americas until 1492. Columbus first encountered native Americans using tobacco for ceremonial and — believe it or not — medicinal purposes. Most of us are so busy laughing at the 1950's commercials claiming that smoking had health benefits that we forget that tobacco was long used to alleviate everything from upset stomachs to headaches.

Wasn't smoke unhealthy for native Americans too? For one thing, it was smoked only in moderation. There were no ten-peace-pipe-a-day chain smokers then, the equivalent to our two-pack-a-day smokestacks. No historians or missionaries ever recorded the deep habitual inhalation of smoke from rolled and lighted tobacco leaves. The pipe was the nicotine delivery system of choice.

Besides using pipes, native Americans placed tobacco in the mouth and inhaled powdered snuff — all practices which persist to this day (in various forms) throughout the world. A Franciscan monk who accompanied Columbus on his second voyage in 1493 documented tobacco's widespread use throughout the New World. He introduced it to the Portuguese court upon his return. The natives were not concocting ways to make the tobacco more addictive, but the demand for the stuff began to grow. The Spanish didn't waste any time cashing in; they were growing tobacco commercially in their West Indies colonies as early as 1531.

27

The "wonder weed" was still confined to the Iberian Peninsula when, in 1559, Jean Nicot brought some to France. This French diplomat at the court of King Sebastian of Portugal gained immortality for carrying an addictive substance across state lines.

The botanical name for the plant, Nicotiana tabacum, and the name of its most important constituent, nicotine, are derived from Jean's surname. Those magic words, "No thanks, I don't smoke," were first uttered in the English language in 1565 thanks to the efforts of Sir Walter Raleigh.

Despite occasional outbursts of protest, tobacco consumption increased wherever it was introduced. Renaissance sailors, like today's baseball players, liked to enjoy tobacco while they worked and idled, and the former did a lot of globetrotting. Tobacco seeds are incredibly easy to transport. Three to four hundred thousand seeds, enough to grow up to four acres of tobacco, weigh just one ounce. A single pod contains over 40,000 seeds. As tobacco use steadily increased, demand led to widespread efforts to cultivate the plant. Tobacco was grown commercially in what is now Cuba and Venezuela by 1580, in Brazil by 1600, and in China, Japan, and South Africa by 1605.

The soil of Virginia and the Carolinas proved to be excellent for cultivation, and for that reason tobacco played an important role in American history, dating as far back as the Jamestown Colony of Virginia in the early 1600's. It was commonly used as a form of currency throughout the American colonies, and in 1775 to 1776 they shipped 100 million pounds to England. Benjamin Franklin secured a loan for the rebellious colonies in 1777 by making a contract with the French tied to 5,000 casks of Virginia tobacco.

During the next century, tobacco was established as an important American cash crop for both international trade and a growing domestic consumption. Unlike today, our early tobacco industry was not dominated by cigarette manufacturers. In fact, several of today's powerful cigarette makers, including Lorillard and R.J. Reynolds, had humble origins as producers of smokeless tobacco.

Cigarettes Roll into History

It may come as a surprise to learn that cigarettes did not arrive as a common commercial product until shortly before the 20th century.

Americans of earlier generations enjoyed tobacco in other forms — they smoked cigars and pipes, inhaled tobacco powder, and used smokeless tobacco. By the late 19th century, an enormous quantity of tobacco was consumed in the United States. With few cigarettes on the scene, 2.5 billion pounds of cigar tobacco were consumed in 1880. Pipe, snuff, and plug (chewing tobacco), added another 150 million pounds of tobacco consumption in the same year.

Smokeless tobacco was favored by the masses because a supply could be carried and conveniently used throughout the day of the typical rural American laborer. Smokeless tobacco was popular at all levels of society. The halls and chambers of the United States Congress contained spittoons as late as the 1930's.

We think of a reporter or telephone repairman working with a cigarette dangling from his lips, but smoking in its early days was a job in itself. Before cigarettes were mass produced they had to be hand rolled. Loading a pipe or clipping a cigar required almost as much work as keeping the darn things lit. Chemicals that keep paper and tobacco burning evenly had not been developed, and safety matches were not available. Until the turn of this century, smoking tobacco of any type was considered a time-consuming leisure activity.

Cigarettes originally had none of the glamour that Hollywood gave them. In fact, they were made from crushing scraps of tobacco left over from manufacturing other products. This gave cigarettes a second-class image, so cigarette smoking was relegated to the lower classes, immigrants, and a few dandies. In fact, only 500 million cigarettes were consumed in 1880.

Cigarettes Were an Accident Waiting to Happen

If cigarettes were such a minor tobacco product in 1880, how, by 1924, did cigarette consumption surpass chewing tobacco? The dregs-to-riches story of cigarette supremacy is a classic American success story — complete with its tragic medical aftermath in our own time. The story involves happy accidents, great social movements, technical innovations, and good old fashioned Madison Avenue selling — factors which were largely in place by 1890.

An accident made cigarette smoking more intensely pleasurable and dangerous. In 1839, an attendant monitoring the heat (or flue) curing of Virginia bright leaf tobacco fell asleep. The tobacco was accidentally over-cured. It was presumed that the batch of leaf was ruined.

Instead, however, the tobacco was found to be very flavorful and light smoking, allowing for deeper inhalation and maximum pleasure. Somehow, life often seems to charge a price for physical pleasures. With this deep inhalation came an increased tendency toward tobacco addiction and all the medical ills that we have come to know.

In 1864, a strain of tobacco called White Burley was planted near Higginsport, Ohio. It was subsequently discovered that this leaf had the exceptional ability to absorb additives up to 25 percent of its weight. This gave cigarette makers the capacity to throw in additives and to blend tobaccos for optimal smoking characteristics.

The increasing urbanization of America indirectly contributed to the rise in popularity of cigarettes. In 1882, a German physician by the name of Robert Koch discovered the bacterium that causes tuberculosis. It was soon ascertained (correctly) that this germ could be carried from one individual to another through close contact, and it was further postulated (incorrectly) that spitting tobacco juices was a likely route of infection. This put an immediate stigma on chewing tobacco, and it was soon shunned in "polite" urban society. Ironically, the healthier smokeless tobacco was considered unsanitary, and cigarette smoking was erroneously seen as the healthier alternative. Smoking grew in popularity, and smokeless tobacco was no longer king of the hill. Today's medical facts may permit reversal of this historical irony, allowing smokeless tobacco to regain its popularity while dangerous cigarettes fade into obscurity.

Wars played an important role in the spread of tobacco and cigarette use. During the Crimean War in the early 1850's, French and English soldiers were introduced to Turkish and Russian tobacco blends and cigarettes. Philip Morris, an English tobacconist, capitalized on this by producing cigarettes with these exotic tobacco blends for British and American markets in the 1850's and 1860's.

During the American Civil War, Union soldiers made cigarettes from Virginia tobacco, marching home with a taste for these easily inhaled, high nicotine domestic blends. Tobacco has long been one of the necessities of war, perhaps because it has provided harried soldiers with a pleasant diversion, an emotional lift, and the reduced ability or desire to taste army food. During the Revolutionary War, George Washington, perhaps to prevent all Virginia tobacco from being shipped to France, issued the following plea to the Continental Congress: "I say, if you can't send money, send tobacco." Cigarettes were considered to be effective for dealing with the stress of trench warfare in the First World War. They were given to soldiers in 1917 and 1918, and General Pershing pleaded with Americans at home, "Tobacco is as indispensable as the daily ration; we must have thousands of tons without delay."

In the Second World War, American soldiers again received free cigarettes in their rations. Several manufacturers, recognizing the vast future market, went to great lengths to provide adequate supplies to the troops. The combined effects of both world wars created millions of nicotine-addicted men. Shortly after the fall of Germany in 1945, with the Central European economy in ruin and no stable monetary system, cigarettes became a widely accepted form of currency. Many American servicemen, even several United States congressmen, benefited handsomely from black market distribution of American cigarettes at that time.

Cigarettes could never have knocked smokeless tobacco off the hill without key technical innovations in manufacturing. Until 1880, all cigarettes and cigars were hand rolled. The added time and higher cost kept the number of consumers down. Then, in 1884, James Bonsack built the first successful cigarette rolling machine, enabling these "little coffin nails" to be mass produced. The graph below illustrates the explosion of cigarette use before and after mass production.

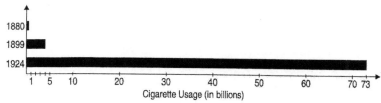

Cigarette Usage (in billions)

Another technical development was perfectly timed with the mass production of cigarettes. The technical difficulties of keeping tobacco lit were solved by 1892 with the successful development of the safety match. Portable fire became available for the first time to the common man, becoming a key factor in the growth of the common man's smoke. Only four years later came the first match box advertisement, and a new marketing era was born. In addition to the development of safe, dependable matches, cigarettes were also manufactured with another big advantage — they only needed to be lit once. (Some of the chemicals that provide this increased combustibility have turned out to be possible toxins.)

Unlike cigars and pipes, cigarettes provided a steady dose of tobacco which burned smoothly and consistently. Instead of being the least convenient form of tobacco enjoyment, cigarettes became the most efficient nicotine delivery system. In our push-button nation whose population is accustomed to instant gratification, the cigarette smoker who wants to live longer should adjust to a convenient alternative (no lighter is needed for snuff) that enters the bloodstream a bit more slowly.

We learn about the robber barons in American history, but we never hear about the tobacco kings who built up the cigarette industry while building themselves massive fortunes. James B. Duke, the future benefactor of Duke University, was no less a talented entrepreneur than J.P. Morgan (General Electric and United States Steel) or John D. Rockefeller (Standard Oil). Between 1880 and 1900 Duke consolidated almost all United States tobacco production, distribution, and marketing into one gigantic corporation, the American Tobacco Company. First, he established absolute control over the mass production technology by obtaining exclusive rights to the Bonsack machine. Throughout the 1880's Duke perfected old strategies for marketing cigarettes and invented new ones. For example, he may have been the first promoter to subsidize the construction of signs for retail merchants, an advertising method still used today by soft drink makers. By 1890 Duke controlled most cigarette production and sales. Between 1893 and 1899 American Tobacco consolidated the important smokeless tobacco market, ending with one of the most well known brands, the fabled Bull Durham. Duke's tobacco empire grew until 1911, when the United States Court of Appeals ordered its dissolution under the statutes of the Sherman Antitrust Act of 1890 (the Standard Oil monopoly suffered the same fate that year).

During the first part of this century a trio of entrepreneurs made significant contributions to cigarettes' increasing popularity Richard Joshua Reynolds founded the R.J. Reynolds Tobacco Company, which introduced perhaps the first truly national cigarette brand, Camel, in 1913. The year of Joe Camel's birth also witnessed the founding of the organization that is now called the American Cancer Society. The legacy of Reynolds' successful career in tobacco remains even today as an important part of the giant conglomerate RJR Nabisco, Inc., one of the nation's largest cigarette manufacturers.

George Hill was a marketing genius who made a previously little-known brand of cigarettes, Lucky Strike, into a household word. By 1926 this brand had captured twenty percent of all United States cigarette sales. In 1927 Hill teamed up with Albert Lasker, considered to be the founder of modern advertising, to break the taboo against women smoking. They focused an advertising campaign for Lucky Strikes directly at women with the slogan "Reach for a Lucky instead of a sweet," which resulted in even higher sales for the brand.

In the 1930's and 1940's, Hill intensified and diversified his tobacco promotion efforts, investing heavily in radio advertising and sponsoring popular entertainers such as Jack Benny, Ethel Smith, and Frank Sinatra. Lasker ironically took a different path in the 1940's. Burned out by the advertising industry he helped establish, he set up a foundation to distribute medical research grants and awards, and with his wife Mary, was instrumental in the reorganization and financial restructuring of the American Cancer Society. The Lasker Foundation Awards for outstanding medical research have been considered among the nation's most prestigious honors.

You can see how the advertising wizards of Madison Avenue had unimpeded access to the American consumer for four decades. Cigarettes became associated with everything from pleasure and sophistication to youthful vigor and success. You have probably heard the furor over some of the early advertisements which claimed that cigarettes were good for one's health. We now know that cigarettes have allowed the health of millions to go up in smoke.

Hollywood helped cigarettes become popular as a symbol of American culture. Smokeless tobacco products had no way to compete for the hearts and pocketbooks of the American public. Cigarettes were mass produced and distributed inexpensively, and were accepted as the most convenient, hygienic, and attractive way for Americans to enjoy tobacco. They were easy to smoke and carry around, and had little effect on other activities. Snuff was not yet packed in neat and discreet pouches, and distribution and advertising of such products was not at all competitive.

With the addictive quality of nicotine keeping loyal customers coming back for more, cigarettes were the perfect consumer product. The only minor problem, which was not recognized for several decades, was a tendency to kill the devoted customer after many years of faithful consumption.

Conspicuously absent thus far from this thumbnail history of tobacco use are any protest movements comparable to the prohibition of alcohol. Tobacco has not been immune from such criticism, although prior to the last three decades the carping tended to be based on moral or religious grounds.

King James I of England published *A Counterblaste to Tobacco* in 1605, just one year after authorizing the famous version of the bible which bears his name. He called smoking "a custom loathsome to the eye, hateful to the nose, harmful to the brain, dangerous to the lungs, and in the black, stinking fume thereof, resembling the horrible Stygian smoke of the pit that is bottomless."

Kings can be politicians, too; James dropped the rhetoric, picked up tobacco excise taxes, and made a bundle for the English treasury.

Do you think Prohibition just applied to alcohol? In 1899, twenty years before the Big Booze Blockade started, Lucy Page Gaston went on a crusade to ban cigarettes throughout the country. She was a success in the conservative Midwest, where cigarettes were banned, albeit temporarily, in Arkansas, Indiana, Iowa, Kansas, Minnesota, Nebraska, North Dakota, Oklahoma, South Dakota, Tennessee and Wisconsin.

How Smoking "Became" Unhealthy

The ravages of smoking appear only after decades of puffing, so medical detectives were slow to pick up on the trail of death and destruction. In 1921 Dr. Moses Barron from the University of Minnesota picked up a clue — he noted an unexplained increase in lung cancer. Further evidence trickled in very slowly. In 1930 German researchers found a statistical correlation between smoking and cancer. By 1938 Dr. Raymond Pearl at Johns Hopkins University had indicted cigarette smoking as life-shortening. In 1950 the smoking gun was found; reports in both the British and American medical research literature confirmed the link between lung cancer and smoking. *Reader's Digest* blazed the trail for the nation's media; in December 1952 it published "Cancer By The Carton." Twelve years later the Surgeon General issued his verdict: Smoking kills.

The cigarette companies have maintained their innocence for three decades, but the trial has placed them — as well as their customers — squarely on death row. Review the evidence yourself in the next chapter.

~ ~ ~

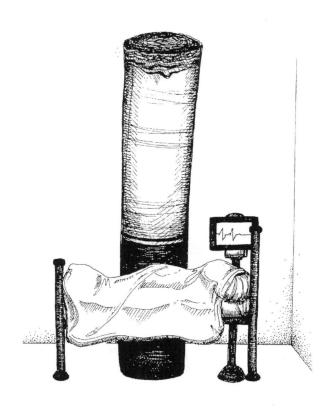

Chapter Three
Cigarettes May Break Your Favorite
Habits
(Like Breathing)

Chapter Three
Cigarettes May Break Your Favorite Habits
(Like Breathing)

Veni, Vidi, Vici
(I came, I saw, I conquered)

> — Attributed first to Julius Caesar,
> this appears on the Philip Morris coat of arms
> on every pack of Marlboro cigarettes.

The Real Price of Cigarettes: Smoking and Health Risks

Cigarette smoking is directly related to as many as 419,000 deaths in the United States annually. It is the single most important avoidable cause of death, directly responsible for the demise of nearly one in five Americans. The toxic, disease-causing combustion products in inhaled tobacco smoke quickly pass through the lungs into the bloodstream, reaching all parts of the body. The graph below illustrates a partial breakdown of the annual death toll of diseases related to smoking.

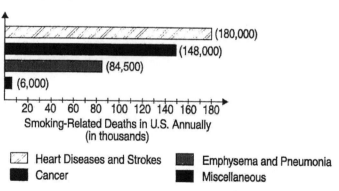

Smoking-Related Deaths in U.S. Annually
(in thousands)

▨ Heart Diseases and Strokes ▥ Emphysema and Pneumonia
■ Cancer ■ Miscellaneous

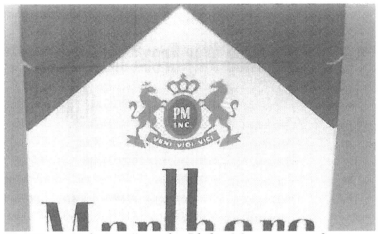
"Veni, Vidi, Vici" on the Philip Morris coat of arms

A little knowledge is dangerous. Are you one of those smokers who knows a little bit about health from your readings and dismisses any dangers of lung cancer because no one in your family has it? Statistics may permit you to be slightly less concerned about lung cancer, but there are throat and other cancers to consider.

Even more importantly, check that family tree for coronary and pulmonary problems (two other categories in the graph above). If you've really asked about both sets of your uncles, aunts, and grandparents, it is unlikely that your genes are so good that nobody in the family has suffered or died from these killers.

Then, if you shrug off the fact that Uncle Herman was 70 when he succumbed to a heart attack and Aunt Thelma was 80 before she contracted pneumonia, ask yourself if these people were heavy smokers. Before you casually dismiss the numbers and fall back on your optimistic chances of surviving to a ripe old age, have your heart and lungs checked. You might be shocked to learn that, medically speaking, your 38-year-old body is already housing vital organs that are "older" than those of old Herman and Thelma.

When you were a sophomore on spring break you might have declared that you wanted to die young — but you probably outgrew that attitude as you grew older and became a spouse, parent, or grandparent. In fact, over one-third of the deaths attributed to smoking occur in people younger than 65 years of age. If a smoker dies of a smoking-related illness, he or she will have lost an average of fifteen years of life. Because these smokers die at an age when they are still active workers and consumers, the economic costs are substantial.

Cancer — "Cigarette" Begins With the Big C

Thirty percent of all cancer deaths are directly attributable to cigarette smoking. Smoking is associated with cancers that develop in airway structures that come in direct contact with smoke, such as the mouth, throat, voice box, and lung. The pollutants flow through the bloodstream to places as far removed as the pancreas, bladder and kidney. The following table is a partial list of the new cancer cases each year in the United States that are specifically related to smoking.

Smoking and Cancer	
Site	New Cases Each Year
Lung	145,300
Mouth	27,400
Voicebox	10,300
Esophagus	9,000
Pancreas	9,600
Bladder and Kidney	27,800
Total:	229, 400

Epidemiologists are getting better at keeping records of all this carcinogenic carnage. It will come as a surprise to no one that over 145,000 new cases of lung cancer occur in smokers every year. Remember that the five year survival rate for lung cancer ranges only from 11 percent to 13 percent. The first reports linking lung cancer to cigarette smoking were published over 40 years ago, so there is no way to claim ignorance. Nationwide each year, more than 2 million years of life are lost prematurely due to lung cancer. How can we be so sure that cigarettes are really to blame?

39

The lifetime risk of lung cancer in nonsmokers is 1 percent, while the lifetime risk in smokers has been reported to be as high as 30 percent. Read these numbers and believe them — insurance companies do.

Other cancers also take their toll. Of the 12,600 new cases of cancer of the larynx each year, over 80 percent are associated with smoking. Eighty percent of deaths from esophageal cancer are blamed on smoking. Smoking is responsible for 50 percent of bladder and kidney cancer deaths in men, and there is an association of smoking with pancreatic cancer and leukemia.

Another type of cancer — affecting the mouth — deserves a closer look. Up to 90 percent of oral cancer is due to smoking. Over 27,000 cases of mouth cancer are seen each year in smokers. These figures on oral cancer have not been fully assimilated by the public or, for that matter, by many health professionals. The common misconception is that lung cancer is the only adverse effect of smoking or, at least, the only place where cancer is a risk.

Oral or mouth cancer, on the other hand, is wrongly associated only with smokeless tobacco use. The misperception arises because tobacco makes real contact with the mouth in smokeless applications. But smoke permeates the lining of the entire mouth (just as it does clothes, drapes, carpeting, etc.), placing cigarette smokers at much greater risk for mouth cancer.

Circulatory Disorders — What Goes Around...

Although it is less commonly known by the general public, smoking also causes a considerable increase in risk of death from heart and circulatory diseases, which are responsible for nearly half of all deaths (1 million) in the United States every year. Of the 90,000 heart attack deaths per year attributable to cigarette smoking, 35 percent occur before the (retirement) age of 65. If you are taking cigarette breaks at work and dreaming about retirement, consider quitting smoking as the single best thing you can do for those post nine-to-five years.

Whatever affects the old ticker and blood circulation can affect that all-important command center in the brain. There are approximately 400,000 strokes annually in the United States, 50 percent to 55 percent of which are directly related to smoking.

Nicotine creates a mild increase in heart rate, but nicotine itself is not directly associated with heart disease. Not so the tar found in cigarette smoke, which is linked to heart and arterial problems. Furthermore, the carbon monoxide produced by smoking leads to faster development of angina, the chest pains related to heart disease. We all wince (or begin to cough) when a truck or bus fills the air with carbon monoxide, and we all fear being in a closed garage where a car has been idling for several minutes; but when smoking we are taking in that same noxious gas, only in small and flavored doses that mask the poison. It might take years of smoking or breathing passive smoke to equal the five minutes in a carbon monoxide-filled garage that is widely known to kill human beings, but each puff of tobacco smoke adds up. We have all heard of despondent people committing suicide in such a smoke-filled garage. Now ask yourself how much you want to drag on those carbon monoxide sticks we call cigarettes.

Heart Disease

While directly linked to lung disease and a number of cancers, smoking plays a more indirect and subtle role in raising the risks of heart disease. Many other factors besides smoking play supporting roles in the development of these problems, but the effect of smoking is unquestionably a big factor. So many smokers have lifestyles that include high consumption of fatty foods, insufficient exercise, and higher than average alcohol intake that, admittedly, researchers find it hard to isolate the smoking factor from the smoker factor. If this book helps you switch from cigarettes to smokeless tobacco, then you will hopefully recover the lung power to do some more exercise and build up the will power to eat and drink with moderation. All of these combined may lower your susceptibility to heart disease.

Heart diseases kill about 1 million Americans every year; this amounts to about fifty percent of all deaths in the United States. Many cases are the result of complications of atherosclerosis, which is a thickening of the walls of arteries leading to partial or total blockage of blood circulation. The development of atherosclerosis and heart disease is very complex, and it is clear that there are many factors beyond tobacco smoke which are important. Given the scope of this book, it is not possible to offer a comprehensive discussion of all the causes of heart disease. I will instead provide a broad overview of these factors.

The key contributors to heart disease can be divided into three general groups: (1) Factors you can do nothing about; (2) those that are partially controllable; and (3) those that you can change.

1. There are several factors that are completely out of your control. The first is your family history. If either of your parents developed heart disease before they reached the age of 60, then you are more likely to develop heart problems too. Asking about uncles, aunts, and grandparents will also help you establish any patterns in your side of the family The development of heart disease in parents older than 60 is not a strong risk factor, since normal aging can involve heart complications.

In addition, there are other genetic factors, such as a specifically inherited trait for unusually high cholesterol levels, which are seen in some families. There are also prominent gender differences in heart disease risks; men are far more likely to die of coronary disease than women. The protection from heart disease that women enjoy is probably related to high estrogen levels during childbearing years. After women reach menopause, their chance of heart disease eventually reaches the level of men.

Race and ethnicity can also be as inescapable a risk factor as old age. In the United States, death rates from coronary heart disease are higher in blacks, probably related to the increased prevalence of high blood pressure in that population. A typical Eastern European high cholesterol diet puts one more at risk than a Mediterranean diet, where olive oil and wine combined with lower cholesterol foods result in low coronary disease figures. Diabetes represents another independent risk factor for heart disease.

2. There are several risk factors that can be partially altered. The first is hypertension, or high blood pressure. The risk of heart disease is higher with hypertension, and strokes are a common problem when high blood pressure is untreated. Some studies have shown a reduction in deaths from heart disease when high blood pressure is lowered through medication.

People who are obese or overweight by more than 20 percent over their ideal body weight are at double the risk for heart disease. Even the location of that extra body fat seems to be important, as those with excessive abdominal fat are in the highest risk group. (So start burning that belly fat and stop burning those cigarettes.)

3. Finally, there are several factors which are under your control. One of the most important controllable (except for specific inherited disorders) factors is your blood cholesterol level. Since cholesterol is transported mainly in molecules called low density lipoproteins (LDL's), these have been considered the "bad" blood lipids. The best single predictor of risk for heart disease is the ratio of "good " and "bad" lipids to total cholesterol. If your doctor alerts you to a problem in this area, it is your responsibility to change your diet. An honest listing of the foods you eat will probably be asked of you right after your doctor determines how many cigarettes you smoke a day.

A couch potato lifestyle with little exercise is another factor in heart disease that is under your control. Exercise increases general fitness, lowers body weight, and lowers cholesterol while raising the concentration of "good" blood lipids. It can also lower the viscosity of the blood, making it less likely that a blood vessel will develop a clot, and it may lower blood pressure. Many people believe that they have to engage in a strenuous athletic program to achieve these benefits. But studies have shown good results from mild exercise three times a week for a total of one hour. Don't worry about aerobics or the health club, take the cigarette out of your mouth and do some vigorous walking.

Your diet can also substantially alter your risk of heart disease. It is possible to reduce blood cholesterol concentrations by at least 20 percent by limiting saturated fats in the diet. Current suggestions include limiting the proportion of dietary fat to 30 percent of your total calories and limiting the proportion of saturated fat to 10 percent of your total caloric intake.

Your doctor or dietitian will help you cut down or eliminate the more dangerous parts of your diet, and the right changes can have a positive effect on the old ticker. Several studies show that for every 1 percent reduction in blood cholesterol, there is a 2 percent decrease in the risk of heart disease.

What if you are already diagnosed with heart disease? Should you eat and smoke like there's no tomorrow? Absolutely not. Other studies have shown that reducing dietary fat will benefit people who already have heart problems. The progression of heart disease appears to slow and there is even evidence that subtle reversal of atherosclerosis is possible.

Smokers are not only notoriously bad eaters and exercisers, but they tend to be bigger drinkers of alcoholic beverages. Heavy beer or booze drinking is notoriously unhealthy, but a little alcohol can be good for you. As has been widely publicized, drinking the equivalent of one or two glasses of wine a day does appear to lower the risk of heart disease. Since alcohol is an addictive substance, health professionals cannot prescribe it as a method of controlling heart disease when many of the other strategies discussed here are equally or even more effective.

While smoking may compound the negative effects of other unhealthy habits listed above, we must try to isolate the issue of tobacco and heart disease. There is general agreement that smoking is an independent risk factor in the development of heart disease. The risk of atherosclerosis increases in proportion to the number of cigarettes smoked. There is even evidence that smoking low tar and nicotine cigarettes, or those with filters, has not appreciably altered heart disease risks. This points to the harmful quality of cigarette smoke as opposed to tobacco or nicotine itself (see Chapter Five).

Equally important is the fact that when people quit smoking, their risk of heart disease drops quickly. In as few as three years the former smoker's risk of heart disease is the same as that of someone who has never smoked (with all other risk factors being equal). Even smokers who have suffered a heart attack have a 10 percent to 40 percent increased survival rate if they quit.

Smokeless tobacco contains plenty of nicotine, which has immediate effects on the circulatory system. These include a mild increase in heart rate and a transient increase in blood pressure. Still, there is no clear evidence that nicotine by itself is directly related to heart disease. It is obvious that the smoke which causes breathing difficulties is also related to straining the cardiovascular system that involves the action of the heart and circulation.

There are many other components of cigarette smoke which are potentially harmful. For example, the tar component of cigarette smoke contains an enormous number of free radicals, an especially reactive group of molecules derived from oxygen. There are at least 10^{14} free radicals present in every puff of cigarette smoke. These molecules have been implicated in the development of atherosclerosis, heart disease, cancer, and emphysema.

Smoking also produces high levels of the carbon monoxide we discussed above. This chemical compound is poisonous because it decreases the amount of oxygen that the blood can carry to the tissues. Do you want to know why so many smokers seem to have poor stamina for exercise? Studies have shown that high carbon monoxide levels can accelerate the lack of oxygen available to the heart during a workout. This same slow choking off of necessary oxygen leads to faster development of angina, or the chest pain related to heart disease.

If you are starting to become confused about what exactly in cigarettes causes heart disease, you are not alone. After thousands of research studies, about the only clear message is that all of the factors that we have discussed play some role, with different factors being more important for different individuals. Because there is so much overlap between these heart disease factors, it is better to take a case-by-case look at each smoker. When forced to generalize about smokers, one must assume that they are more likely to consume too much dietary fat, to exercise with less frequency, and to have higher cholesterol levels than nonsmokers. If you are one of those smokers with the guts to quit or switch to smokeless tobacco, then you might also be motivated to modify these other risk factors.

As a matter of fact, after you switch to smokeless tobacco you'll even be able to swim or play tennis or team sports while keeping the juices flowing with tobacco enjoyment. Just try doing the butterfly stroke with a cigarette!

Now hold on there. What about smokeless tobacco use and the development of heart disease? Within the past two years a couple of studies regarding this issue have come from Sweden (the smokeless tobacco capital of the world). In the first, published in 1992, the effect of smoking and smokeless tobacco use on the development of heart attacks was studied. The results showed that smoking resulted in an increased risk for heart attacks, while smokeless tobacco use carried no risk. In a second study published in 1994, smoking and smokeless tobacco use were studied as risk factors in deaths due to heart disease and cancer among construction workers in Sweden. This study showed that smokeless tobacco use carried some risk for dying from heart disease in men who were between 35 and 54 when the study started. Most importantly for this book, the recorded risk for users of snuff was much smaller than for those who were either light or heavy smokers. In fact, the risk in smokeless tobacco users was the same as smokers who had quit from one to five years previously. In older men, who were ages 55 to 65 when the study started, there was no heart disease risk related to smokeless tobacco, although the risk related to smoking was still present. This study also reported the interesting but contradictory finding that smokeless tobacco use was associated with no cancer risk. (This is inconsistent with most other studies, as I'll discuss in Chapter Seven.)

Admittedly, possible problems in the interpretation of the 1994 study include the effects of other risk factors. For example, it is common in studies such as these to control for the effect of dietary fat and blood cholesterol, since these have been shown to be higher in smokers than nonsmokers and may influence the apparent effects of smoking or using smokeless tobacco. This effect is called "confounding." In other words, smokers may have diets higher in fat, or they may have other lifestyle differences which may account for some of the higher heart disease rates. Unfortunately, the effect of these other important components was not studied. In the study published in 1992, the important factor of serum cholesterol was shown to be the same for people in the healthy and unhealthy groups. Again, it is extremely important to point out that all tobacco use carries some health risks. However, regarding heart disease, it appears that *switching to smokeless tobacco is as beneficial as quitting smoking.*

What counts for you, then, is the fact that smokeless tobacco use carries fewer risks for all diseases than smoking, including the next category, lung disease.

Lung Disease — When Breathing Is a Drag

Smoking is also responsible for a large percentage of deaths from lung disease. The Centers for Disease Control and Prevention (CDC) has estimated that smoking is directly responsible for over 84,500 deaths annually from pulmonary disease including emphysema, asthma, influenza, and pneumonia. Over 80 percent of the 70,000 deaths per year from emphysema alone are related to smoking.

Emphysema presents a special problem for smokers. It involves a slow distension of the air sacs of the lungs, followed by the destruction of the partitions between these spaces. The lungs become filled with air, but because of the disintegration of the air sacs, the air cannot be pushed back out of the lungs.

The signs and symptoms of emphysema are not pleasant. Because the destruction of the air spaces is a gradual process, the affected individual experiences worsening breathlessness with each new exertion. The condition becomes so severe that it is eventually impossible to walk across the room or even sit up in a chair. Because air cannot be moved in and out of the lungs efficiently, there is insufficient exchange of oxygen and carbon dioxide. The skin takes on a blue color from this lack of oxygen in the tissues. Circulation is affected, with swelling occurring in the hands and feet.

Emphysema is one of the most crippling of all diseases related to smoking. As lung destruction progresses, the unfortunate individual slowly suffocates. Quitting smoking at the onset of serious emphysema is too little, too late. Once the damage occurs to this extent, it is irreversible.

Have I scared you? I hope so. You are probably more inclined to listen to a doctor with verifiable statistics than to your loving, but nagging, spouse or friend. Now the good news. I am not advocating going cold tobacco turkey for you diehard smokers who would rather die hard than quit. I'm merely asking you to get your same tobacco buzz in a different way. A way that will give you added years of health and life — perhaps enough time for your damaged vital organs to stage a recovery.

What Are You Really Paying For Cigarettes?

I don't mean to ask if you get a good deal on cartons of Marlboro's at your local carryout. In the currency of time, every year of life and health is priceless. A study I completed with Dr. Philip Cole at the University of Alabama at Birmingham shows that, on average, the 35-year-old American man who smokes will lose almost eight years of life. Of course, the eight years are a mathematical entity. Some lucky individuals will live to 95, smoking three packs of unfiltered Camels a day. Then again, many poor souls will die in their forties or fifties after battling lung cancer or during a sudden, severe cardiac arrest. Those smokers who get picked off early by the cigarette sniper lose around fifteen years on average.

We are human beings, not averages. But smoking certainly stacks the deck in favor of the house — the funeral home, that is. You'll be happy to know that you can enjoy tobacco pleasure and not lose those theoretical eight years if you switch to smokeless tobacco.

The number crunchers have also come up with some figures as to what smoking is costing the country in terms of Medicare expenses. Joseph A. Califano, Jr., head of Columbia University's Center on Addiction and Substance Abuse, puts the bill for hospital expenses stemming from substance abuse at $20 billion annually. Yes, cigarettes are figured in, and they account for a whopping 80 percent of the total. By contrast, illicit drug abuse accounts for merely 3 percent, with alcohol abuse chipping in only 17 percent.

Cigarette smokers who don't drink are likely to look down on alcoholics, but let them learn a little humility when they discover that sick smokers are costing the nation over four times as much as sick drinkers. The smokers don't share the alcoholics' frequent liver problems, but they do have the lion's share of lung cancer, coronary artery disease, and chronic lung diseases (see above).

Women are catching up to men among these Medicare patients, as the "You've come a long way, baby" generation comes all the way to 65 or older.

Yes, the rise in numbers of people who have quit smoking helps keep these figures under control, but Califano claims that hospital Medicare bills will still cost Americans $1 trillion over the next twenty years — and smoking will continue to be the single largest contributing factor (to the tune of $800 billion).

Whether or not these astronomical figures are correct (see below), the younger Americans who have to foot these bills are going to get mad at smokers for more than secondhand smoke. It's another good reason to put out that cigarette and put that discreet pouch of smokeless tobacco between your cheek and gum.

Smoking's Costs — Another Perspective

Even though I have come to bury cigarettes, not to defend the industry, a few words are in order to counter the antitobacco hysteria. Too much of the one-sided crusade against tobacco would have tobacco users solely responsible for all of the nation's health care bills. The $800 billion figure cited above is supposed to be tobacco's share of Medicare costs due to abuse of tobacco, alcohol and drugs.

In 1994 alone, we are to believe that $16 billion of Medicare's hospitalization expenditure may be blamed on Joe Camel and his flock. No wonder that all this scapegoating (scapecameling?) is leading to threats of further "sin taxes" against tobacco users! The American public must think it only fair to tax to oblivion these national threats to the economy.

But the charges that smoking drives enormous health care costs deserve another look. It is true that smoking-related illnesses account for over 400,000 deaths (about 20 percent of the total) a year in the United States. These deaths, granted, are not cost-free to our healthcare system, but let us imagine what would have happened if those individuals did not smoke. They would not have died of a smoking-related illness, but, a few years later, these older men and women would have died from some other cause. Do not forget that even a great many Americans who do not smoke die from cancers and heart failure. The illnesses that they would have died from still would have cost the nation a bundle, but they wouldn't have been charged to the tobacco account.

It is therefore clear that the elimination of all tobacco use will not eliminate our health care bill. Age is the far greater killer, and the increased longevity of our aging American population guarantees astronomical health bills as we enter the next century. A cynic might even consider that unhealthy practices like drinking and smoking that kill off 50- or 60-year olds before they become 80-year olds is a boon to the nation's economic welfare. The point is that aging and mortality drive our health care financial problem — not smoking.

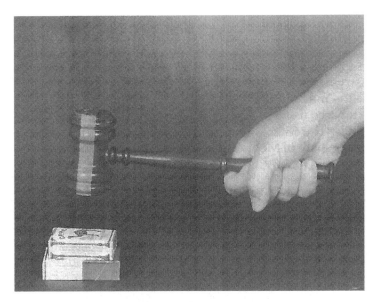

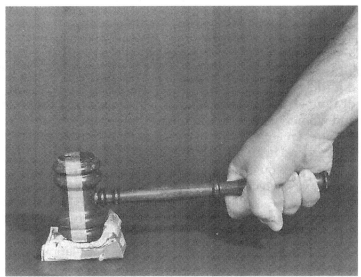

The judgement on cigarettes

In a 1989 study published in the *Journal of the American Medical Association*, researchers at the University of Michigan and the RAND Corporation assessed the many costs not borne by the smoker or his family. These external costs to be paid directly or indirectly by others in society include sick leave, disability compensation, insured medical costs, group life insurance, pension, lost taxes on wages, and insured losses from fires. This large tally, after a comprehensive and sophisticated analysis, was then compared to the level of excise taxes then in effect. The study's surprising conclusion: Cigarette smokers pay their way.

The excise taxes on cigarettes more than compensate for the external costs that smokers impose on society's nonsmokers. In fact, the actual costs were calculated at fifteen cents a pack, and federal and state excise taxes actually added up to 32 to 37 cents a pack. If fairness and objective truth reigned supreme, you wouldn't have had to hear all this from me for the first time. Too many health care experts and the politicians they have in tow are happy to pin our mismanaged health care crisis on the tobacco industry. Because they have targeted an industry rather than a particular product, cigarettes, much of their attack will wrongly include smokeless tobacco. The problem of cigarette smoking requires the bold, practical approach (smokeless tobacco) that is raised here. It is too bad that the national crusaders against tobacco, like all lynch mobs, are not particularly subtle or discriminating.

Nonsmokers should not feel too smug, for their favorite vice may be just around the corner. Let drinkers be informed that the same test above found that the drinkers, unlike smokers, are not paying their way. The external costs of drinking were calculated at 48 cents per ounce consumed, while the average excise taxes for distilled spirits, wine, and beer only came to 25, 3, and 9 cents respectively. So, if any drinkers out there are gloating over the way smokers are being treated — watch out! Alcohol is clearly next on the hit list.

Next on our hit list is secondhand smoke, another burning issue which will be history after smokeless makes its comeback.

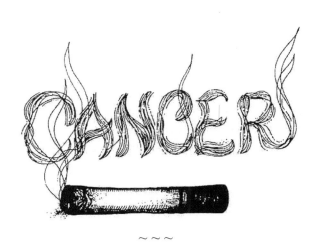

~~~

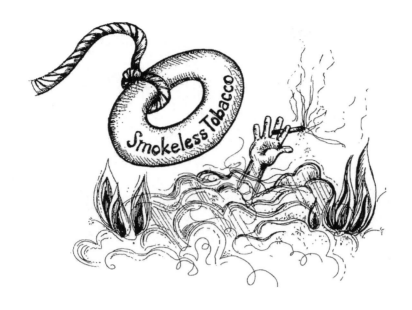

Chapter Four
Secondhand Smoke Is Your Firsthand Problem

Chapter Four
Secondhand Smoke Is Your Firsthand Problem

Bernard Shaw made the pertinent inquiry: "How can the smoker and the nonsmoker be equally free in the same railway car?" This is one of the fundamental problems — that of special and conflicting interests — in this heterogeneous railway car we call a nation.

— Sydney Harris
Publishers Newspaper Syndicate

So far, you have been urged to switch from smoking to smokeless tobacco for your own health. In this chapter you will be urged to quit for the sake of others — the people around you who breathe in your smoke secondhand. Passive smoke is such a burning political and legal issue that every smoker has discovered that smoking in public is now a very inconvenient thing to do.

You probably began smoking for social reasons or peer pressure from teenage friends, but now smoking may make you a social outcast. The antismoking crusaders have yet to make cigarettes as illegal as heroin, but in many cities you will have to be almost as clandestine as a junkie looking for that alley or bathroom stall to shoot up in. Let's look first at the science behind the issue of secondhand smoke.

Are Your Wife and Children Smoking Too?

A recent study in the *Journal of the American Medical Association* renewed calls for tougher measures limiting secondhand smoke after finding that women whose spouses smoke at home have a 30 percent excess risk of developing lung cancer than women with nonsmoking husbands. These women never took a puff themselves, yet they had this higher lung cancer risk simply because of the smokers they lived and worked with.

In this case-control analysis which studied the effects of passive smoke, 653 female lung cancer patients who never smoked were compared to a control group of 1,253 women without lung cancer. As bad as the 30 percent excess lung cancer risk was from secondhand smoke at home, this risk was higher if the women also had exposure to passive smoke at work. At home, these women were able to manipulate the ventilation, and to ask their spouses to confine smoking to certain areas. This cannot be done in a smoke-filled workplace or social situation where fans, air cleaner systems, or ionizers are rarely used. Women who worked in smoky offices exhibited an excess lung cancer risk of 39 percent, and those regularly exposed to secondhand smoke in social situations registered an increase of up to 50 percent.

Parents who smoke may also be placing their children at risk for respiratory problems. Children up to age five have been studied most often, and mothers who smoke are especially implicated because they spend more time with the preschoolers. Asthma is the most common lung problem in children, affecting 2 to 5 million youngsters nationally. Studies of children with asthma have shown that secondhand smoke affects lung performance and increases the sensitivity of the airway. Mothers who smoke have children with higher rates of asthma and possibly earlier onset of symptoms than nonsmoking mothers. Although earlier studies have relied on questionnaires, a 1993 study in *The New England Journal of Medicine* measured nicotine breakdown products in children's urine. This provided evidence that secondhand smoke is directly related to these pulmonary problems.

Young children may be susceptible to more than lung damage. The New York University Medical Center conducted tests with baby chicks who were exposed to passive smoke for sixteen weeks. These young birds had significantly higher deposits of fat, cholesterol and other artery-clogging substances in the aorta than a control group with an identical diet but with a smoke-free environment.

Could Smoking Create Fat and Cholesterol?

The experiment focused on the particular vulnerability of young living things to secondhand smoke, with the findings serving to warn us about human infants. The study, however, appears also to implicate environmental tobacco smoke in the production of life-threatening fat and cholesterol, an area that deserves more research. Up to now, scientists have assumed that smokers are simply well represented in the groups of people who eat the unhealthiest foods, but this study suggests that smoking and cholesterol may be more than common lifestyle traits. These factors may interact in the blood vessels to enhance the chances of life-threatening complications.

Medical researchers in Boston found it easier to estimate links between heart disease and passive smoke than lung cancer and passive smoke. They believe environmental tobacco smoke to be responsible for 32,000 deaths from heart disease. A presentation at the World Conference on Lung Health in Boston put secondhand smoke in third place as the nation's leading cause of preventable death. In second place was alcohol abuse, while in first place, of course, was firsthand smoking.

The American Heart Association (AHA) has also warned of the cardiovascular damage caused by breathing someone else's tobacco smoke. In a recent position paper, the AHA estimated some 40,000 deaths a year from heart and blood vessel diseases that occur as a result of passive smoke.

Living things without lungs can also register toxic effects from the thousands of chemicals and forty known carcinogens contained in secondhand smoke. Passive tobacco smoke has recently been shown to have a witheringly toxic effect on plants.

Plant abuse! Wait a minute. Time for a reality check. The debate over secondhand smoke has gotten somewhat out of control. As you'll see later in this chapter, the regulators, legislators, and litigators have jumped on the secondhand smoke problem, stretching the data far beyond what is reasonable. Despite all of the numbers I cited above, the evidence for secondhand smoke is definitely softer than that presented to the jury for the firsthand variety in Chapter Three. This shouldn't come as much of a surprise.

Secondhand smoke is mainstream smoke diluted over 100,000 times. Because of the dilution effect, only about 100 of the 3,000 chemicals in firsthand smoke have been found in samples of environmental smoke. The National Academy of Sciences estimated that the concentration of inhaled nicotine — one of the most common components of tobacco smoke — is 57,000 to 7 million-fold less for the passive smoker as compared to the smoker.

Where Secondhand Smoke May Be Exaggerated

Without denying secondhand smoke as a possible cause of health problems, there are points to be made here to round out the debate. In all fairness, I must add that the health risks of secondhand smoke are subtle and therefore hard to prove. As I explained for firsthand smoke in Chapter Three, heart disease development is a complicated business, and it is very difficult to distinguish between the effects of secondhand smoke and all of the other contributing factors. Did the long-suffering spouse share the same diet, exercise level, and alcohol intake along with the smoke? Besides lifestyle, factors like family history, sex, advanced age, and other medical problems must be weighed. There are quite a few factors that would increase or decrease a spouse's chances for a heart attack that have nothing to do with how much smoking goes on.

Lung cancer from secondhand smoke is also more tricky than the newspaper reports would have it. Lung cancer among nonsmokers is rare, and doctors and statisticians are often hard pressed to find the cause. Because the number of such cases is small, there is a larger range of possible coincidences when trying to identify the risks. This leads to a larger margin for error. When it is reported that there is a 30 percent excess risk for lung cancer in women whose spouses smoke, the margin of error dictates that the excess risk may indeed be as low as 4 percent. At this level it is virtually impossible to be sure if there is any additional risk of lung cancer in these women.

These statistical limitations were discussed in the *Journal of the American Medical Association* report, and they indicate that lung cancer in "passively" smoking women is far from a certainty. As so often happens with reports of medical research, the fine print revealed the real message. The subtle implications of this study would have been much harder for the general public to grasp.

Even though these points would have injected necessary balance into the antismoking hysteria, they were apparently not newsworthy enough for the press releases.

Let the spouses of smokers lose a little less sleep over the secondhand smoke in their homes. There are problems to deal with, but probably not so severe that only a divorce will fend away lung cancer or heart disease. The nonsmoking wife of a smokestack spouse has enough to be concerned about, such as impending widowhood.

The tobacco companies' counterattack in the press picked up on the weakness of the passive smoking charges. On June 28, 1994 Philip Morris took out ads in the major papers, running the provocative headline: "How Science Lost Out to Politics on

Secondhand Smoke." At least the ad was frank about the tobacco companies' own guilt in setting themselves up for a lynching by the media. The cigarette makers were compared to the boy who didn't cry wolf. That is, the manufacturers had been so consistent with their blanket denials of the link between cancer and smoking that no one believed them when they (truthfully, this time) denied the strong links between passive smoke and cancer.

Adjusting Science to Fit Policy - The EPA Report

The regulators at the United States Environmental Protection Agency joined the antismoking frenzy in 1992 with a report entitled "Respiratory Health Effects of Passive Smoking: Lung Cancer and Other Disorders." The report concluded that "widespread exposure to environmental tobacco smoke in the United States presents a serious and substantial public health impact." Furthermore, the EPA has ruled that secondhand smoke causes 3,000 lung cancer deaths per year in nonsmokers in the United States, and it has designated secondhand smoke as a "Group A" carcinogen.

Although it has been hailed by tobacco opponents as a landmark study, the scientific credibility of the study has been challenged recently. For example, in order to arrive at the "proper" conclusions about secondhand smoke, the EPA investigators, in the words of one official, "engaged in some fancy statistical footwork" to synthesize the "indictment." According to John C. Luik of The Niagara Institute, there is evidence that two recent studies on the effects of secondhand smoke were purposefully excluded because they were not supportive of the EPA's conclusion, and other studies were misrepresented in the analysis. Nor was the EPA deterred from its antismoking mission by unbiased personnel. It stacked the working group and advisory board with known tobacco opponents, and it ignored internal criticism of the report by its own scientists. Finally, to label secondhand smoke as a "Group A" carcinogen, the EPA had to violate its own guidelines for assessing agents as possible carcinogens.

As carefully documented as these criticisms are, they have gone largely unnoticed. Instead, the EPA report has served as a catalyst for other interventions.

The Legislative Push Against Human Air Pollution

The House Subcommittee on Health and the Environment passed the Smoke-Free Environment Act in May 1994, which was designed to ban smoking in most public buildings except bars, restaurants, prisons, tobacco shops and private clubs. Further congressional consideration of the bill was terminated by the November 1994 elections. Antitobacco crusader Henry Waxman from California was replaced as subcommittee chairman by Virginian Thomas Bliley, who is unenthusiastic about sweeping federal regulations of the tobacco industry.

The bill was gathering supporters, such as the McDonald's Corporation, which banned smoking in all 1,400 corporate-owned restaurants. In addition, 90,000 other restaurants like Dunkin' Donuts and Hardee's jumped on the bandwagon to stop you from that habitual after-meal cigarette or cigar. Associations of office managers and building owners would also have joined in to make your cigarette breaks at work a thing of the past.

Although federal efforts have waned with the Republican-controlled Congress, the cities of Los Angeles, San Francisco, and New York, along with the states of Vermont, Maryland, Washington, California and Utah have already adopted strong workplace smoking bans. The legal activity was set into motion by the 1992 report from the Environmental Protection Agency that declared passive smoke to be a "known human lung carcinogen." This wording followed a more moderate assessment than the American Medical Association report, suggesting that the spouse of a smoker had only a 19 percent greater chance of getting lung cancer.

A smoker can no longer shrug and say, "Well, it's my life." The secondhand smoke issue has made smoking a matter of everyone else's life. Activists point to secondhand smoke as a health hazard that kills Americans every year, and the American Lung Association regards cigarette fumes as a leading indoor source of air pollution.

A cigarette smoker who switches to smokeless tobacco not only clears his or her conscience about harming others, but also avoids all the social and legal hassles that come with producing passive smoke. And don't think antismoking legislation is a fad that will go away as quickly as it came. No-smoking laws increased tenfold in the 1980's. Some of the more famous smoking bans involve public schools and military bases. It all began with Minnesota's landmark Clean Indoor Air Act back in 1975. Restrictions went sky-high in 1988 when the United States Congress banned smoking on commercial airline flights of less than two hours. This ban has since been extended to all domestic flights. A bag of peanuts won't help your nicotine addiction, so you better consider smokeless tobacco.

By 1991, 44 states and the District of Columbia had restricted smoking in public areas, promoting a smoke-free environment for 80 percent of the United States nonsmoking population, compared with 8 percent only two decades earlier. In March 1995 the tobacco-growing state of Maryland joined California, Vermont, Utah and Washington in banning smoking in most workplaces, excluding bars and restaurants. In April 1995 New York City's Smoke-Free Act went into effect. The law bars smoking in office buildings, stadiums (Yankee and Shea included), movie theaters and other public places. But the hottest debate centered around the dinner table, because the law stubbed out after-dinner smoking in restaurants seating more than 35 people. That includes 11,000 of the Big Apple's 15,000 eating establishments.

What restaurants, hotels, ballparks, and airlines ought to do, for both their nicotine-addicted clients and their patrons who are concerned with secondhand smoke, is to have smokeless tobacco products available. Of course, sale to minors should be prohibited.

Even with these restrictions, approximately 50 million adults over age 35 are still regularly exposed to environmental tobacco smoke. More importantly, 50 to 70 percent of all children in the United States live in homes with at least one adult smoker.

This book's smokeless tobacco plan is not only the most workable solution for this smoky mess, but it most fits the American ideal of preferring freedom of choice over intrusive government regulation. The smokeless tobacco solution is market-based. You, the consumer and smoker, are in control. You can still exercise your constitutional "pursuit of [tobacco] happiness" without harming others and without requiring an act of Congress to force your decision. If enough smokers switch to snuff very soon, we could watch the cigarette join the phonograph in our museums. If any further legislation might be needed, it would be to stiffen the penalties for selling addictive substances to minors. Yes, that means all tobacco products.

Legal Problems With Secondhand Smoke

The Circuit Court of Dade County in Florida has been hearing a class-action lawsuit filed against the tobacco industry by 30 flight attendants. They want compensation for damages done by secondhand smoke inhaled in airplane cabins over many years of service. The price tag of these damages — $5 billion! Now you get an idea why your workplace is probably smoke-free or will be soon. Your company might even be run by a chain-smoker, but no one is going to let a business go up in legal smoke.

A proposal to ban coffee in the workplace would set off riots. But even those who have sworn off caffeine don't claim any damages from coffee aroma. While someone might mind the smell of coffee, and employers certainly mind many long coffee breaks away from one's workstation, no one minds if an employee or coworker is chewing gum or using smokeless tobacco.

You might take the side that the EPA's study was full of "fancy statistical footwork," and you might even be an enraged smoker who feels that your constitutional rights are being endangered. Nothing will help. The majority of concerned nonsmokers are alarmed about risks — proven or unproven — from breathing secondhand or passive smoke, and they are more than willing to use legal measures to challenge the nation's sacrosanct "pursuit of happiness" in the process.

Unless you live in a private, single-family home, the new, aggressive laws against smoking could even catch up to you as you smoke under your own roof. Just ask the Conrad family of Dover, New Jersey. They had to go to court when their upstairs neighbors complained about nausea, coughing, aggravated asthma, and allergy symptoms from the Conrads' smoking. The neighbors even charged that the smell of tobacco smoke had permeated their carpets and bed linens. The judge in this case was lenient, ordering the upstairs neighbors to get a smoke-eater device, but this case is a warning to all smokers.

If you are a confirmed smoker, you now sense that the government, your employer, and even your favorite restaurants and stores are out to get you. As for me, I'm only out to get you to switch tobacco products. There is no smoke involved in putting a pouch of snuff between your cheek and gum. You suspect that it's not the same as puffing on that after-dinner cigar or dragging on that cigarette at work — but you don't know until you try it. You can and will get all the nicotine satisfaction you want. And you should be satisfied to know that employers, colleagues, neighbors, and fellow sports fans and travelers will no longer be concerned about being downwind of you.

Once you find the smokeless tobacco product you like best, you'll be delighted to know that you can even satisfy that nicotine urge while in close quarters like elevators, the car-pool, and church.

"May I Smoke?"

You hear the courteous question more these days, but not as often as you might expect when considering how passive smoke is a "well-established" health hazard. The tobacco industry would like common courtesy to solve the problem of environmental tobacco smoke — not annoying legislation. However, studies show that smokers' courtesy is not all that common.

Only 47 percent of 22,000 smokers surveyed in 1989 said that they light up a cigarette indoors without asking people around them for permission. The message of passive smoking is gaining momentum, however; the 33 percent who said that they don't smoke indoors around others is up 4 percent since 1978. A whopping 80 percent of all nonsmokers consider smoking to be harmful or annoying, yet only 4 percent tend to ask the smoker to stop. The number of aggressive nonsmokers is bound to rise, as the vast majority of Americans now know that it is harmful to breathe in the smoke of others. One can expect the most militant responses, of course, from those millions who have quit smoking.

Death or Taxes

Besides hitting the smoker with laws to protect innocent bystanders, states are increasing cigarette taxes that hurt the pocket of even the lone smoker. As can be expected, the tobacco states of North Carolina, South Carolina, Kentucky, and Virginia only tax a pack of cigarettes to the tune of 2 to 7 cents. States like California, Connecticut, Hawaii, Minnesota, New York, Rhode Island, and Washington all tax a pack of cigarettes at 33 cents or more per pack.

Will this patchwork of high and low state taxes help? Not as much as you might think. The different taxes in various states — and in Mexico and Canada — will only encourage cigarette smuggling from lower tax areas. The experience of our northern neighbors represents a great example of the disastrous consequences of indiscriminately raising tobacco taxes. Starting in the late 1980's, the Canadian government escalated cigarette taxes by about fivefold. By 1993 cigarettes cost $4 more in Canada than in the United States, and there existed an enormous smuggling industry worth an estimated $5 billion with net profits of $300 million. Seventy percent of smuggled cigarettes were channelled through Akwesasne, a Mohawk reserve near Cornwall, Ontario.

Early in 1994 it became obvious that the federal Canadian government was incapable of dealing with the effects of its ill-conceived tax hike. Although antismoking activists were outraged, the Canadian prime minister introduced a plan to cut the federal tax by $5 per carton, with an offer to match further cuts by provinces of up to $10 per carton. This story should serve as a warning to those who would propose sweeping policy changes to deal with tobacco use.

Moreover, the addiction to nicotine is so strong that most smokers will grumble and reach deeper into their pockets. Higher costs may have some benefits, however, in deterring young people on limited budgets from taking up the tobacco habit. Anything that cuts down the number of new tobacco addicts is a good thing. Of course, lawmakers need to know that smokeless tobacco is a part of their solution, not a part of the cigarette problem, if they care for the health of their constituents.

The latest volley fired by the army of antismokers involves a $2 tobacco tax and the "Campaign for a Million Lives." According to the Coalition on Smoking or Health, a $1.76 tax increase would result in approximately seven million fewer smokers — saving an estimated 1.7 million lives. The campaign has the ears of Congress and the backing of former Surgeon General C. Everett Koop, former President Jimmy Carter, and some 100 different organizations. Death and taxes are inevitable, and so are more taxes to combat smoking deaths. Unfortunately, levies on all tobacco products are being considered. If lawmakers read this book, they might consider sparing smokeless tobacco to give smokers a way out. The bottom line here is not crushing the tobacco industry, but saving lives; and switching from cigarettes to snuff will save lives.

What's Wrong with these Pictures?

On June 21, 1994 the R.J. Reynolds Tobacco Company fired a full-page advertising volley in the New York Times and other papers in its ongoing media counterattack. Two-thirds of the full-page spread was dominated by four photos of people: smoking; drinking an alcoholic beverage; drinking coffee; and eating a hamburger. The respective captions beneath the four photos read: "Some politicians want to ban cigarettes"; "Will alcohol be next?"; "Will caffeine be next? "; and "Will high-fat foods be next?"

Although from an obviously biased source, the ad may have a point about the politically correct police and which pleasure they will strip us of next. But the tobacco executives are forgetting a major difference between cigarettes, coffee, alcohol, and fatty food. That difference is the focus of this chapter: the perceived danger to others. The caffeine fiend and the burger king are forcing nothing negative or harmful on the people around them. Yes, the alcohol abuser can be dangerous, especially behind the wheel. Indeed, alcohol may be next on the list, but although smelling a drinker's breath from a foot away may not be pleasant, it is not going to take away even a minute from your life expectancy.

Beneath the photos and captions in the ad appears the headline in bold print: "Today it's cigarettes. Tomorrow?" The copy below discusses the campaign by the Food and Drug Administration, the Department of Labor, and Congressmen who are attempting to prohibit smoking in America. These groups are accused of proposing a tax increase of up to 800 percent, which will price cigarettes out of existence. They are also singled out for "introducing regulations that could lead to a total ban in private as well as public places."

In case the flag-waving appeal to American rights and privileges isn't clear, it is spelled out in the next paragraph's line about "threats to the freedom we enjoy in our society." The cigarette industry is attempting to say that legislation curtailing the threat of passive smoke is the greater danger, although antismoking groups counter with their right to breathe smoke-free air in public places. Bernard Shaw's railway car is getting more crowded, but you have to hope that the engineer can keep the train on the track.

The smokers in a tightly enclosed railway car, airplane, or room are forcing their fumes on others. The ad, however, only considers how the "prohibitionists" intend to "force their views on the whole country." The ad goes to extremes to warn us about these crusaders who may go on to ban books, movies, and music — bringing up the picture of Nazi-style book burnings. There is even a reference to the threat to "cholesterol 'addicts'" — as if high-fat foods required tolerance and involved withdrawal symptoms.

The ad appeals to smokers and nonsmokers to settle their differences peacefully. The ad's tagline calls for "accommodation" and courtesy between smokers and nonsmokers but nowhere hints at the best compromise of all: smokeless tobacco. Americans would never consider banning snuff, whose aroma is less pervasive than coffee, and which may be safer for the body and soul than fatty burgers and demon rum.

In their follow-up volley to the major newspapers (on June 28, 1994), the R.J. Reynolds people filled a full page with pictures of a bar, a truck, and a private home with a service person on the way in. The text of the ad referred to proposed legislation that would ban smoking in any building used by ten or more people at least once a week (except in a specially ventilated smoking room), in private vehicles (even when alone), and in private homes when a delivery or service person was present. According to the tobacco company, "Government control or government intervention" is the issue here, not the possible harm from passive smoke.

How Many Unwanted Cigarettes Are Too Many?

A month earlier the R.J. Reynolds Tobacco Co. had put out an advertisement (New York Times, May 23, 1994) which directly tried to counter the significance of secondhand smoke. The company claimed that, on average, the person exposed to environmental tobacco smoke would only take in the equivalent of smoking one-and-a-half cigarettes per month. This figure, though hard to prove, would indicate an exposure too small to correlate to illnesses like lung cancer. But the RJR people are missing the point!
Nonsmokers do not want to breathe in any smoke, and they are demanding zero cigarettes per month exposure when in public.

Where There's Smoke, There's Fire

To measure more accurately the devastation from smoking we must also hear from firefighters around the country. According to the National Fire Protection Association, each year in this country 1,300 people perish in fires set by burning cigarettes. I am not just talking about a few smokers who fell asleep and burned themselves as their beds went up in flames. I am including all the innocent people who die in buildings, brush fires, and industrial accidents because every cigarette is potentially a lit fuse, to say nothing about the property damage that drains insurance companies and personal fortunes.

Tobacco officials took some heat from this issue as well in the Congressional hearings of spring 1994. The president of Philip Morris was asked about making paper cigarette tubes that were less of a fire hazard. The executive responded that those cigarettes were harder to draw smoke through and did not taste as good. When children die from the deadliest kind of secondhand smoke — smoke inhalation from a cigarette fire — we should not be concerned with smokers' comfort and taste. Good taste and much easier breathing can be obtained from using smokeless tobacco.

No fire was ever started with the consumption of smokeless tobacco. Nicotine addicts who have switched to snuff do not have to worry about their ubiquitous books of matches and cigarette lighters that invite disaster from curious little hands. Certainly, there are no secondary victims in the use of snuff tobacco — especially the form that I recommend for men and women, business people, and professionals.

You'll never burn someone while walking or gesticulating with a pinch of tobacco in your mouth, and with no burn marks or ash droppings to worry about, you're not likely to ruin someone's furniture or designer suit. Of course, to get to the point of switching to smokeless tobacco, you have to be concerned about how good you look on the inside of your body.

Cigarettes' Glamour Is Gone

If I'm going to end a chapter on secondhand smoke with an aesthetic point, let me remind you how you started with cigarettes in the first place. You looked good smoking, or so you felt. Your heroes in the movies, the cowboys on the billboards, that suave lady executive who came a long way, baby — and, of course, the people in school that you emulated — looked so cool lighting up, dragging in, letting smoke curl through their lips and nose, flicking off the ash...

Well, I have news for you: It's the nineties. The glamour days of George Hill and Albert Lasker (see Chapter Two) are gone forever. Rather than images of movie stars, nonsmokers are more likely thinking: "Look at that insensitive smokestack. Don't come upwind of me with those dangerous fumes. Wonder why that person was too weak to quit? Guess you can't teach an old dog new tricks."

Calling all smokers insensitive and weak is not only inconsiderate but also terribly inaccurate. In the next chapter I'll explain why tobacco's iron grip is so strong. Because once you understand why it's so difficult to quit smoking, you'll be ready for the smokeless tobacco solution. Compared to the promiscuous chemical exhaust of cigarette smoking, a tiny pouch of snuff is no more visible or obnoxious than a breath mint or a lifesaver. Many healthy years later, you'll see that the switch to smokeless tobacco was for you and those around you, indeed, a life saver.

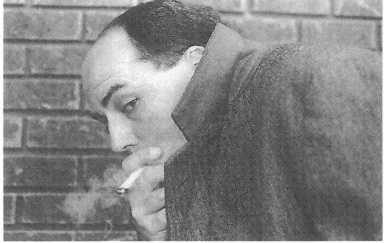

The alley smoker, stealing a quick cigarette before returning to the office

~ ~ ~

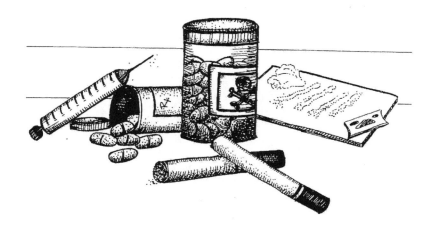

Chapter Five
Nicotine Is the Captor, But Smoke Is the Killer

Chapter Five
Nicotine Is the Captor, But Smoke Is the Killer

*Tobacco, divine, rare, superexcellent tobacco, which goes far
beyond all the panaceas, potable gold, and philosopher's
stones, a sovereign remedy to all diseases... but as it is
commonly abused by most men, which take it as tinkers do
ale, 'tis a plague, a mischief, a violent purger of goods,
lands, health, hellish, devilish and damned tobacco,
the ruin and overthrow of body and soul.*

— Robert Burton (1577-1640)

When tobacco is burned, the resulting smoke contains a rich mixture of many chemicals. In fact, as many as 3,000 separate chemicals have been identified! Many of these are the dangerous carcinogens and toxins that are responsible for the diseases detailed in Chapter Three.

Nicotine is one of the most abundant constituents of smoke. I will review the evidence that nicotine is a potent and addictive drug, but everything you read about the effects of firsthand and secondhand smoke in this book does not refer to the burning of nicotine. It is important to stress that nicotine itself has not been linked to lung damage of any kind, nor has it been conclusively tied to the myriad of cardiovascular problems exhaustively studied by doctors and researchers around the globe. Finally, nicotine is definitely not a cancer-causing agent. I cannot emphasize strongly enough that the problem with smoking primarily involves the other 2,999 chemicals produced when tobacco is burned. In other words, it's the cigarette's "delivery system," not the nicotine. With tobacco products on trial as killers, remember that it is predominantly the cigarette that is the smoking gun.

When you smoke tobacco you are doing a lot more to your body than taking in nicotine or even burning tobacco. Health experts have recently intensified their demands that cigarette makers release lists of the many additives found in their products. Many chemicals in cigarettes (which are not found in smokeless tobacco products) have been added to help the tobacco and cigarette paper ignite and stay lit.

In the words of Gregory Connolly, the director of tobacco control for the state of Massachusetts, "The additives are essentially there to make smoking easy, to help a blowtorch turn a young lung into rice pudding." Toxicologists are concerned about the combustion products of chemicals like the insecticide methoprene, which have never been studied. Dietrich Hoffman, associate director of the American Health Foundation, comments that the ingredients of cigarettes "are approved as food additives, but when you add them to tobacco and burn them you may form toxic or carcinogenic agents."

Understanding Nicotine

Smokers derive a lot of pleasure from smoking tobacco. You may be reading this book because you or your loved one actually enjoys lighting up a cigarette and taking several deep puffs. A smoke may be especially welcome when you are in a stressful situation or when you need to relax, or you may enjoy smoking when you need to concentrate on a difficult problem at work or at home. Cigarette smoking can activate that mental pressure-relief valve, which is followed by the feeling that the problem can be solved, and the crisis will pass. These feelings are real and not just a figment of your imagination.

Many tobacco opponents claim that these sensations are not truly pleasurable, but are merely the satisfying of induced cravings and avoidance of withdrawal symptoms. One of the big advantages of the smokeless tobacco solution is that it addresses either view of smoking equally well. That is, it doesn't matter if you are a smoker who is unwilling to quit because you enjoy tobacco, or if you are unable to quit because of nicotine craving and withdrawal. In either case you recognize the potential life-shortening effects of this nicotine delivery system, and the smokeless tobacco solution can work for you.

Most of the sensations related to smoking are a direct result of your body's reaction to nicotine, a fascinating and misunderstood drug found only in tobacco. Let's take a detailed look at what nicotine is — and what it is not.

Nicotine is a product found naturally throughout the tobacco plant. It is most plentiful in the leaves, where it can make up between 5 and 10 percent of the plant's weight. The nicotine content varies considerably among the many strains of tobacco. As cigarettes are often "blends" or mixtures of several different types of tobacco, careful attention must be paid to the overall concentration of nicotine in the final products.

Nicotine is absorbed in different ways, depending on the type of tobacco used. For example, when cigarette tobacco is burned, nicotine exists within the tobacco smoke in a form that cannot be absorbed readily in the mouth or nose. Thus, cigarette smokers must inhale deeply into the lungs, where nicotine is able to quickly pass across thin membranes into the bloodstream. Once in the blood, the effects of nicotine are felt almost immediately. After the cigarette is finished, however, nicotine levels in the bloodstream fall fairly quickly. Smokers commonly want another cigarette within an hour.

In contrast, nicotine is contained in smokeless tobacco products in a form that is readily and efficiently absorbed through the lining of the mouth. It is not necessary to swallow tobacco juice to absorb nicotine. In fact, nicotine is not absorbed effectively in the stomach. When using smokeless tobacco products like snuff, the nicotine reaches your bloodstream a few minutes later than with smoking. More than compensating for this relatively minor delay, the nicotine level in your blood remains high for a much longer period of time than it does with a cigarette.

This means that you won't have to use smokeless tobacco as frequently as you smoke. If you switch to snuff, therefore, you not only save the agony of serious cardiovascular and pulmonary diseases, but you also save some serious pocket change on the difference between larger numbers of cigarettes and the lesser amounts of smokeless tobacco necessary to keep nicotine flowing into your bloodstream. Many successful switchers in my quit smoking program now use only one or two cans of snuff per week instead of two packs of cigarettes a day. At about $2 per pack of cigarettes or can of snuff, these switchers have reduced their weekly tobacco bill from $28 to $4.

Nicotine is absorbed in amounts which are subconsciously yet very carefully regulated by the smoker. Studies have shown that you are remarkably efficient in maintaining your individual nicotine comfort level throughout the day. You probably have very low nicotine levels when you wake up in the morning; in order to get that

71

level up to your comfort zone, you may smoke several cigarettes early in the morning. Chances are that you smoke at fairly regular intervals throughout the rest of the day to maintain that desired level.

Variations in smoking patterns can occur in response to changes in daily routine, stress levels, or the availability of cigarettes. This last factor has become increasingly important as smoking is banned or severely restricted in most enclosed public places. When you have to leave your desk and building to smoke a cigarette outside, you are probably smoking more intensely (with longer and deeper puffs) to get your daily nicotine needs out of fewer cigarettes. It is highly debatable whether these smoking restrictions are helping you quit or reducing your exposure to deadly toxins.

Let's look at a great example based on clinical studies. If you are a two-pack-a-day (40 cigarettes) smoker and you are only allowed five cigarettes a day, you will get several times as much nicotine from each cigarette as you normally do, which only decreases your total daily nicotine intake by half. No problem at all if you're only restricted to fifteen cigarettes a day. With harder and longer puffing, fifteen can equal 40!

What about those filtered and low tar, low nicotine products? They are really effective, right? Wrong — and here's why.

The United States and Canadian governments have sponsored tests of nicotine and tar concentrations in cigarettes since 1967. A common misconception is that these tests determine the amount of tar and nicotine in the tobacco itself. This is not true. Instead, these tests employ smoking machines that puff on each brand of cigarettes in a systematic fashion so that the nicotine and tar "yields" can be measured and compared between brands. The results of these tests are seen on every cigarette package and advertisement. But these tests have little resemblance to reality, because as a smoker, you may unconsciously manipulate and defeat the best intentions of the so-called "safer" cigarettes, which include filters and designs which are supposed to dilute the smoke.

Let's examine the facts and fallacies behind these safer cigarettes. Filters were introduced soon after the Second World War, at the time when the health effects of smoking were just starting to surface. The Kent brand of cigarettes employed filters in 1952, but two years later it was clear that the filters were too efficient. That is, smokers were not able to get any pleasure (i.e., nicotine) from smoking Kent cigarettes. In 1954, the filters were "improved" by making them less efficient. Two decades later filters had captured the market, and smokers breathed a sigh of relief — as did the cigarette makers. They were putting out a "safer" product ("Because we really care …"). Additionally, the filter material was cheaper than tobacco, and filter cigarettes use 15 percent less tobacco than those without filters ("...about our profits").

Cigarette makers also decreased tar and nicotine yields by punching tiny holes in cigarettes, thereby increasing the air flow through the cigarette during puffing. The more air brought through the cigarette, the less smoke from the burning tobacco and the less tar and nicotine. In principle this sounds like a great idea. However, cigarette smokers have found that by curling their finger around the cigarette near the filter, they can block the air holes and defeat this design feature, thus increasing the available nicotine (and toxic tar) per puff.

So don't bet your life on these "safety" features, because they have probably had very little effect on either your smoking patterns or the resulting health risks. That is because you get the nicotine you want despite these safeguards. You may get your fix by puffing more frequently and more intensely. If you've switched from higher yield to lower yield cigarettes, studies show that you consume more nicotine than predicted by the smoking machine tests.

In fact, studies even show that smokers of high yield nicotine cigarettes consume less nicotine than predicted. Thus, the nicotine and tar yields as determined by the government tests are very poor indicators of how much you actually absorb.

Nicotine is a drug which produces many more effects on you than you ever imagined. It is such an active drug that virtually no system in the body is left unaffected, but the main effects occur in the brain and the circulatory system. These effects are summarized in the table on the next page.

As the table illustrates, nicotine's major effects are centered in the brain. It is interesting to note that nicotine is a close match for some human brain cell receptors, because nicotine's chemical structure is similar to naturally occurring substances that affect the brain. That is why it can affect your appetite, act as a stimulant, or enhance your concentration and performance on certain tasks. In addition, I'm sure you have experienced a sense of well being and an upturn in your mood after smoking. Nicotine also has the effect of stimulating the breathing center within the brain.

Effects of Nicotine on the Body
Brain: Stimulant
Enhances concentration
Enhances performance
Sense of well being
Mood elevation
Stimulates breathing center
Circulatory: Increases heart rate
Increases blood pressure
Constricts blood vessels
Other: Increases free fatty acids
Increases catecholamine release
Increases saliva and lung secretions

The brain may even be involved in nicotine's effect on the circulatory system, resulting in both a higher heart rate and blood pressure. However, it is very important to point out that these increases are only seen while nicotine is present in the bloodstream; both the heart rate and blood pressure return to previous levels afterward. In fact, the blood pressure of smokers is on average equal to or lower than that of nonsmokers. Cigarette smoking does not primarily cause high blood pressure; however, high blood pressure and smoking are a dangerous combination.

I have listed the other effects primarily to demonstrate that nicotine touches virtually every system in the body with widely diverse results. Free fatty acids are a product of the breakdown of body fat which is in storage. Catecholamines are hormones that are produced in the adrenal gland. Their release may activate many other processes which are important in your response to mental and physical stress.

How Badly Do You Need Cigarettes?

Nicotine is addictive. Do you or your loved one think that this book may not be relevant to you because you are not a hard-core cigarette smoker? You don't have to be a pack-a-day smoker to be addicted. Let us find out with a few easy observations if you are indeed dependent on the nicotine found in cigarettes.

You probably started smoking when you were a teenager. At the time, it was the cool thing to do. If you are over 30, you probably did not even hear much in the media that convinced you that smoking would become an incredibly powerful addiction as well as a health danger "in the long run." A few tobacco executives are even claiming today that cigarette addiction cannot be proven — but the medical community has established data that cannot be ignored.

Even though you have thought about quitting and/or have seriously tried quitting in the past, you haven't been able to shake the "habit." Mere habits are not that hard to break. The signs of true addiction can be more subtle than you think. Remember that there are thousands of cocaine, alcohol, and medication-based addictions out there that are vehemently denied by otherwise intelligent substance abusers.

If you are truly hooked on cigarettes, chances are that many of the following now apply:

1. You smoke at least a pack of cigarettes a day. (Count them all, including your routinely non-routine cigarette breaks.)

2. You smoke cigarettes with regular nicotine and tar levels. (Don't dismiss this as brand loyalty. See if your Camels and/or Trues are adding up to a certain dosage.)

3. If you have tried or now use low nicotine, low tar cigarettes, you find yourself smoking more often, or, when smoking, you are drawing on the cigarette more heavily or more frequently (Ask a close associate to confirm your response.)

4. You smoke your first cigarette immediately after you wake up; you smoke more during the first two hours of the day than during the rest of the day.

5. You find it increasingly frustrating to not be able to smoke in public places. Consciously or not, you avoid smoke-free environments and people you've marked as antismoking.

6. You smoke even if you are ill and in bed and about the same on work days and days off.

If you have responded in the affirmative to at least some of these profile points, then, my friend, you don't have a cigarette habit. You have a true nicotine addiction.

While it is important to define nicotine addiction for the purposes of this book, it is even more important for the definition not to be socially judgmental. I am not condemning you any more than I would a caffeine addict (commonly called a coffee or cola drinker). I am not trying to be negative with you at all. I am only trying to motivate you towards some positive modifications in behavior that I believe you will find to be refreshingly satisfying.

Tobacco use is not yet a crime, but the addictive qualities of nicotine warrant a comparison to drugs like heroin. Just as heroin addicts get treatment with methadone maintenance programs (see the Introduction), we must be bold enough to offer smokeless tobacco (a safer, more acceptable delivery system for nicotine) to millions of cigarette smokers. The smokeless tobacco solution, like methadone maintenance, is scientifically sound but will generate a lot of controversy based entirely on inappropriate and condescending attitudes and beliefs.

It has become far too common for you, a member of a distinct minority (about 25 percent) of the population, to be increasingly labelled by the remaining 75 percent as an unacceptable criminal. It is wrong to stretch health concerns to outright discrimination simply because you are addicted to nicotine. It is true that nicotine is a drug, in the sense that it is a biologically active molecule capable of producing a number of effects after human consumption. However, if objectively evaluated, many things that you and I consume can be considered drugs: from simple foods containing sugars, proteins, and fats to more complex substances like vitamins.

If it helps you shake off any discomfort or stigma, compare yourself to the millions of junk food junkies who are welcomed with dessert trays in restaurants rather than curtly being told that the object of their desire is prohibited. Millions of others are similarly addicted to caffeine, and I can apply the same profile points above to their daily doses of coffee, tea, and/or soft drinks. As a smoker, you shouldn't get too smug about the prevalent caffeine addiction. Remember, medicine has traced many serious illnesses and conditions to the by-products of smoking, not to those of coffee and Twinkies.

Coffee and Cigarettes

Let's look at the caffeine analogy more closely, because it is indeed an addictive drug. Chances are that smokers and nonsmokers alike are hooked. One-half of the World's population consumes caffeine in tea, and another one third get their fix from coffee.

Millions more find daily doses in soft drinks. Caffeine's origin in soft drinks has a botanical basis: caffeine is a component of the kola nut from which Coca Cola was originally derived. However, modern beverages of many brands are purposefully spiked with the drug.

Like nicotine, caffeine is found naturally in plants like tea, coffee, kola nuts, and cacao beans (from which cocoa and chocolate are made). In fact, it is even placed in the same general chemical class as nicotine. But the similarities do not end there. The table below compares the effects of nicotine with those of caffeine.

Similarities of Nicotine and Caffeine		
	Nicotine	**Caffeine**
Brain:	Stimulant	Stimulant
	Enhances concentration	Enhances concentration
	Enhances performance	Enhances performance
	Sense of well being	Sense of well being
	Mood elevation	Mood elevation
	Addictive: Psychic dependence	Addictive: Psychic dependence
	Withdrawal	Withdrawal
	Tolerance	Tolerance
	Stimulates breathing center	Stimulates breathing center
Circulatory:	Increases heart rate	Increases heart rate
	Increases blood pressure	Increases blood pressure
	Constricts blood vessels	Constricts blood vessels
Other:	Increases: Free fatty acids	Increases: Free fatty acids
	Catecholamine release	Catecholamine release
	Saliva and lung secretions	Stomach acids
		Urine flow

The table speaks for itself. As you see, many of the effects that are attributed to nicotine, including those characterizing its addictive nature, are also attributed to caffeine, but coffee, tea, and cola drinkers are not labelled as social outcasts. There are no caffeine-consumption-only sections in restaurants, office buildings, and airports. Caffeine users are not condemned as "addicts," even though by every measure of drug addiction they are. Why not?

The answer is so simple that it is seldom given careful thought. Consumers of caffeine do not suffer health effects that can be easily associated with their addiction. Although caffeine affects almost every organ system in the body, producing (relatively minor and positive) mental and physical effects, it is consumed in a relatively safe manner. How different things might be if coffee beans were ground up, rolled into papers, and smoked to get that "top o' the morning" feeling.

Let's review some specific qualities that make nicotine an addictive drug. First, it produces a strong emotional or psychological need which results in manifest craving of further doses. Second, it creates physical dependence; when nicotine is not available, you start feeling the symptoms of withdrawal, which include restlessness, irritability, anxiety, drowsiness, impatience, confusion, and impaired concentration. There are no powerful convulsions wracking your body, like heroin junkies going cold turkey, but your desire for a cigarette is as intense as the illicit drug abuser's need for heroin or cocaine.

The third characteristic of classical addiction involves tolerance, which occurs when subsequent doses of a drug produce fewer effects. You already know about the tolerance of nicotine's effects: the first cigarette you smoked probably produced dizziness, nausea, and even vomiting. Several cigarettes later, you were tolerant of nicotine's effects.

Nicotine's addiction potential may be enhanced by other chemicals in cigarette smoke. Acetaldehyde, naturally produced in the combustion of sugars and other tobacco leaf components, may make cigarettes twice as addictive as it combines with nicotine.

The Nicotine Addiction "Secret"

To the casual observer of the hearings on the tobacco industry that dominated the nation's print and electronic media in mid-1994, one verdict seems to have been delivered. The tobacco companies appear to be guilty of covering up damaging research that they themselves conducted in the 1960's and 1970's. During those years, research presentations were cancelled, laboratories were shut down, and scientific careers were uprooted — all to protect the dirty secret that cigarette smokers get hooked for life by a powerful addiction to nicotine. The cigarette makers have responded weakly with the fact that many smokers have and continue to successfully quit. This excuse for a defense has not been applied to heroin, another highly addictive substance that thousands have been able to quit.

The nation is rightfully outraged that the tobacco industry has kept this pivotal research hidden for all these years. With 46 million potential clients, the class action legal vultures are circling. Before all the lawyers and reporters swoop down to pick the bones clean, let me place in proper perspective this apparent cover-up issue.

Nicotine addiction is no deep dark secret recently blown out of hiding. In fact, nicotine is one of the most thoroughly studied drugs of all. Only 80 years after Columbus discovered tobacco and the New World in 1492, crude nicotine had been isolated and identified. It was chemically purified in 1828, and the molecular formula of nicotine was determined in 1843. British scientists were describing the effects of nicotine on the nervous system as early as 1889. From the 1930's to the 1950's, many medical authorities already considered tobacco use to be habit-forming or addictive. In 1936 tobacco use was described as "a form of drug addiction, even though a pleasant one, not affecting criminal statistics."

In 1942, L. M. Johnston conducted some remarkable experiments where nicotine was successfully injected into smokers to satisfy their cravings for a cigarette. Johnston reported these findings in the internationally renowned British medical journal *The Lancet*, where he also discussed nicotine tolerance, craving, and withdrawal symptoms. His conclusions: "Clearly the essence of tobacco smoking is the tobacco and not the smoking. Satisfaction can be obtained from chewing it, from snuff-taking, and from the administration of nicotine."

By the 1950's the topic of nicotine addiction had moved out of the medical journals and was published in books for the general public. *The Habit of Tobacco Smoking* (by W. Koskowski, Staples Press Ltd.) appeared in 1955, followed in 1959 by A. King's *The Cigarette Habit: A Scientific Cure* (Doubleday and Co.).

During the 1960's and 1970's, when, according to critics, suppression of tobacco industry research on nicotine was at a maximal level, nicotine "happened" to be the subject of thousands of independent research articles published in the public domain. Medline, the National Library of Medicine's computerized data base, lists 1,000 such studies between 1966 and 1976. The numbers increased to 1,500 in the period from 1976 to 1984, and to nearly 4,000 during the last decade. Many of the research reports published in the 1970's and 1980's were largely scientific validation of what smokers had been saying for nearly a century. These reports, summarized below, should sound very familiar to you by now.

1. The first few cigarettes produce unpleasant side effects.
2. The side effects diminish with each cigarette.
3. Smoking becomes enjoyably pleasant.
4. Daily smoking patterns become predictable.
5. Smoking often continues despite health problems.
6. Withdrawal from smoking is very unpleasant.
7. The abstainer craves a smoke even years after quitting.

The tobacco industry executives used a simple strategy for many years to deal with the insurmountable evidence for the addictive nature of nicotine: denial. The strategy has taken advantage of semantic confusion, as the field of drug addiction suffered bewildering changes of terminology. Over the past several decades, terms like habituation, addiction, abuse, and dependence have been bandied about without a single, uniform definition. By the time the Surgeon General issued the landmark report on smoking in 1964, the World Health Organization had imposed some linguistic order by recommending the term "drug dependence" to replace the more slippery "addiction" and "habituation." In 1980, the American Psychiatric Association finally defined "Tobacco Dependence Disorder" and firmly placed it among other Substance Use Disorders in their authoritative *Diagnostic and Statistical Manual of Mental Disorders III*.

It is now preposterous to deny the reality of tobacco and nicotine addiction. The tobacco companies' denial strategy is largely driven by fears of product liability litigation. But the mass of medical evidence that has accumulated about nicotine also makes it absurd to think that the tobacco industry cover-up of secret research on nicotine addiction is of any significance.

You are probably familiar with the charge that cigarette manufacturers artificially modify the amount of nicotine in cigarette tobacco. Here's another verdict that should be taken to the Common Sense Appeals Court. As I have noted, cigarettes are blended from several different strains of tobacco, the properties of which will also change over time. Thus, it is conceivable that cigarette manufacturers adjust the nicotine concentration to achieve consistency in the tobacco's taste — of which nicotine plays an important role. Even if the amount of nicotine in cigarette tobacco is artificially modified, you cannot deny that a Marlboro smoker deserves the same product uniformity as a McDonald's, Pizza Hut, or Coca Cola consumer.

As I have already discussed, there is an additional and compelling reason to provide cigarettes with consistent nicotine levels: the United States and Canadian governments require disclosure of nicotine concentrations on all packages and advertisements.

We have already seen that smokers are remarkably efficient in regulating their daily nicotine intake, regardless of the amount that manufacturers put in the tobacco. A high nicotine cigarette is not puffed as often or as aggressively as a cigarette with a lower nicotine content or with an efficient filter.

Thus, using high nicotine cigarettes may not raise your nicotine consumption at all. In fact, it may reduce the amount of dangerous smoke you take in. Ironically, as I have noted, light and ultralight cigarettes may increase your exposure to cigarette smoke toxins as you puff on them more often and more vigorously to get the amount of nicotine you are used to. So, instead of a conspiracy to spike higher nicotine content in cigarettes, the real plan to increase consumption may involve the proliferation of the "safer" light brands.

You now know why you are unable or unwilling to quit smoking. However, nicotine has gotten a bum rap by the antitobacco coalition. Not only has it been attacked (correctly, of course) for its addictive potential, but it has also been undeservingly blamed for all of the diseases attributed to smoking. The deliberate confusion of nicotine addiction with health effects has been counterproductive to and has even prevented intelligent discussions of and solutions for the dilemma facing smokers like you.

Nicotine is not the cause of cancers of the lung, throat, mouth, pancreas, bladder and kidney. Much progress has been made in the past 30 years in the ability of scientists to identify chemicals which cause cancer. Many research studies have attempted to prove that nicotine causes cancer: none have been successful. For example, when nicotine is given to laboratory animals in large doses, no cancers are produced. Nicotine is the most frequently studied chemical agent in tobacco for one very good reason — by weight it comprises a substantial proportion of tobacco. Thus, it is the easiest component to measure in tobacco products and cigarette smoke, as well as in the bloodstream of tobacco users.

The Burning Question

If nicotine is not the culprit in smoke that puts you at substantial risk for various cancers, then what is? The answer to this burning question is buried somewhere within the large number of complex chemicals which are produced when tobacco is burned — a total of about 3,000!

Many of these chemicals are produced in tiny concentrations, and they may only exist in an active form for seconds before the body detoxifies them. This makes them virtually impossible to study. Despite their small amounts and transient presence, smoking is an efficient and rapid way to inject these chemicals into the lungs and the bloodstream. Noncarcinogenic nicotine is delivered the same efficient way, but the smoky delivery system makes a cigarette the equivalent of receiving an injection of medicine with an infected needle. This book's argument to switch to smokeless tobacco is really a plea to change over to a safer delivery system.

Let's describe the number of "hits" of cancer-causing chemicals that a typical two-pack-a-day smoker is exposed to. Two packs a day translates into 40 hits a day from the start. If a smoker takes (conservatively) ten drags or puffs per cigarette, the number of doses is 400 per day. Multiplied by 365, the smoker is exposed to 146,000 doses of these chemicals a year. Remember that the latent period for development of smoking-related cancers is twenty years or so. Over twenty years the smoker has had almost 3 million doses! Given these numbers, you might expect that the health effects would be noticeable after only a few years instead of decades. The latent period serves as a tribute to the amazing capacity of the human body to tolerate abuse.

It is clearly the smoke-related chemicals that cause circulatory problems like heart attacks, strokes, and blood clots. True, we have noted that nicotine has effects on the circulatory system, most notably increased heart rate and increased blood pressure. But these effects are temporary, and they are not specifically related to diseases like heart attacks and strokes, the major problems that cause smokers' deaths. As with cancer studies, laboratory research has not proven that nicotine by itself has a significant role in any of these typical smokers' diseases.

You may have encountered studies that accuse nicotine of just these complications. These researchers are throwing out the baby (nicotine) with the bath water (harmful chemicals from smoking). I have studied many scientific reviews of the effects of nicotine on the cardiovascular system, and these reports often confuse unconvincing data about nicotine's effects with much more convincing evidence that cigarette smoke causes higher heart attack and stroke rates.

If nicotine were responsible for circulatory problems, then users of smokeless tobacco, which contains as much nicotine, would suffer from heart disease and strokes at equivalent rates as smokers. However, there is strong evidence that this is not the case. Use of smokeless tobacco carries reduced risks for cardiovascular diseases compared with cigarette smoking (see Chapter Three).

In turning toward the other 2,999 chemicals produced by burning tobacco, one probable culprit definitely worth discussing again is carbon monoxide, the same poison found in abundance in automobile exhaust. It reacts with a molecule called hemoglobin and hinders red blood cells' ability to carry oxygen to your heart, brain, and other vital organs. The heart is called upon to deliver more blood quickly to make up for this oxygen deficit, even as its own needs are unmet. Even more serious is the fact that insufficient oxygen soon causes cells to die. Evidence of this phenomenon is all too common in autopsies of heart attack victims.

Cigarette smoke contains 2 percent to 6 percent carbon monoxide. Everyone living in the industrialized world loses some hemoglobin to carbon monoxide found in the air. However, while the average loss in nonsmokers is 1 percent, smokers lose up to 15 percent. This means that smokers run a much higher risk that vital organs will not receive an adequate oxygen supply, which contributes to higher rates of heart attacks and strokes.

Again, it is the components of the smoke, not nicotine, that are the cause of lung diseases such as emphysema. Lung disorders are attributed to a prolonged inhalation of irritants and toxins. There is no evidence that nicotine is in any way involved in the development of these problems. Each milliliter of cigarette smoke (the volume of about one medicine dropper) contains 2 to 5 *billion* particles of the chemicals that make up the "tar" component of cigarettes. This is what the Federal Trade Commission requires on every cigarette package and advertisement. Remember, there is no tar to list in smokeless tobacco products.

Just like nicotine addiction, we have known about the tar problem for a long time. Back in 1953, Dr. Ernst Wynder and his colleagues at the Memorial Sloan-Kettering Cancer Center in Manhattan showed a direct cause-and-effect relationship between the tar of cigarette smoke and malignant tumors. The backs of mice were painted with the tar extract of tobacco smoke, and 44 percent of the animals developed malignant skin cancer.

A Final Word - The News On Nicotine Isn't All Bad

The devastation of smoking-related diseases has been very closely (and wrongly) associated with nicotine. This has been driven by the deeply held cultural bias of puritanical origin that addictive drugs should not be used for pleasurable or recreational purposes (even though exceptions are still in place for caffeine and, tenuously, for alcohol). Consequently, nicotine was never evaluated judiciously as a bona fide medicine — until recently. Slowly, in medical centers around the globe, researchers are discovering that nicotine may have beneficial medicinal effects in disorders as diverse as Alzheimer's disease and ulcerative colitis.

Alzheimer's disease involves the degeneration and death of nerve cells in the brain, which leads to progressive loss of many mental faculties. The disease exacts a terrible toll on sufferers and their families, but sadly no therapy has proven useful. When nicotine is given to Alzheimer's patients, they show marked improvement in attentiveness and information processing. Nicotine, because of its ability to bind specialized brain receptors, may be unlocking clues to the mechanisms of the illness and may lead to future breakthroughs in treatment.

Even more impressive are nicotine's effects on ulcerative colitis, a disorder of the large bowel. For over a decade it has been recognized that this problem occurs far more frequently in nonsmokers. The onset of ulcerative colitis is sometimes associated with smoking cessation, and a return to smoking may relieve the problem for these people. More recently medical researchers in the

United States and United Kingdom have shown that nicotine delivered by the gum or the patch results in symptomatic improvement and even complete remission of ulcerative colitis.

A similar picture has emerged for mouth ulcers. It has been observed that mouth ulcers are less likely or less severe in smokers and smokeless tobacco users than in nonsmokers. Preliminary reports suggest that this may be due to nicotine, and the drug may prove beneficial in treating severe cases of these painful sores.

Now that the dogma concerning the evils of nicotine shows signs of dissolving, applications for other illnesses are being discussed. A recent balanced and objective medical review entitled "The Beneficial Effects of Nicotine" discussed early research exploring the effects of this drug on Parkinson's disease and sleep apnea.

Is nicotine the next miracle drug? Of course not. Am I prescribing tobacco for mouth ulcers? Not if I want to keep my license. Do I recommend giving snuff to people with a family history of Alzheimer's, Parkinson's, or ulcerative colitis? Not unless they are smokers. Then why is this research important?

These studies suggest that the biases and preconceptions concerning nicotine and nicotine addiction are starting to be shed by forward-thinking scientists. In the investigation of nicotine's effects on the body's normal and diseased states, balance and objectivity are replacing extremism and subjectivity in the nation's research centers. Balance and objectivity are also basic tenets of the smokeless tobacco solution.

~ ~ ~

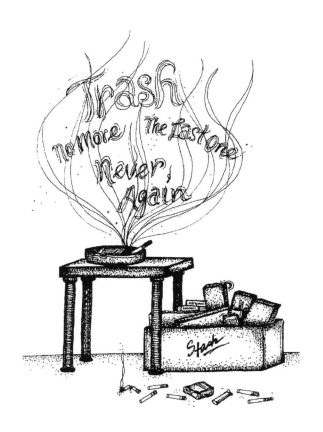

Chapter Six
Stubbing Out that Cigarette - For Good

Chapter Six
Stubbing Out that Cigarette - For Good

To cease smoking is the easiest thing I ever did;
I ought to know because I've done it a thousand times.
— Mark Twain (1835-1910)

Before this chapter discusses some ways to wean you from cigarettes, including a frank review of the failures of many quit-smoking programs and devices, let me offer some positive motivation for quitting. You probably need more than an understanding of the hows and whys of smoking's harm to your body. Before knocking that old familiar friend out of your lips and fingers you need to be convinced that it is not too late to accomplish some good by quitting. If you are an older smoker, you might take another drag on that cigarette with the fatalistic attitude that you can't reverse the long-term damage that you've done. You may have decided to keep on enjoying yourself until you get the two minute warning, but when the score is 56 to 10 against you, the final two minutes of the ball game are irrelevant. If you think losing football players look pitiful on TV, you should personally see the smoker who's been given a diagnosis of lung cancer and three months. Get out now while the score is still tied or you are ahead by a touchdown.

The Handwriting On the Wall Is Legible

A survey of the medical literature on people who quit smoking cigarettes reveals that the health benefits of quitting smoking are quite impressive. They are promising enough to counter the terrible health risks you are taking if you continue to smoke after being warned by your body or your physician. In short, *no matter how old you are or how long you have been smoking*, you can reduce your risk for all smoking related illnesses by stopping *now*.

Cancel Your Projected Chemotherapy Appointment

From the day you quit, you start to reduce your risk for all of the smoking-related cancers discussed in Chapter Three. The risk drops slowest for lung cancer, bottoming out only after twenty years. But at that point, you'll only have 10 percent of the risk compared to your neighbor who kept on smoking. Compared to lung cancer, your mouth cancer risk drops like a lead balloon, reaching the level of nonsmokers in only ten smoke-free years. Esophageal cancer risk also disappears after fifteen years. Other sites in which the cancer risk is decreased by quitting smoking include the pancreas, bladder, and larynx.

Remember that smoking kills more people through heart disease than cancer, so it's great news that the most impressive benefits of quitting are seen in the heart and blood vessels, and with remarkable speed! If you are healthy, smoking cessation rapidly reduces your risk of a heart attack to that of nonsmokers in as little as three years. Even if you have been told by your doctor that you have heart problems related to smoking, you can still reduce your risk of dying from them within a few years after quitting. What if you've already had a heart attack? Don't despair, just desist. Quitting cigarette smoking after a heart attack will give you a 10 percent to 40 percent better chance of surviving. Your risk of having a stroke will fall just two years after tossing away cigarettes, reaching the level of your smog-free friends after five years.

Ceasing to smoke has respiratory and general health benefits as well. Respiratory symptoms such as coughing, phlegm production, wheezing, and shortness of breath may get better immediately. If you have emphysema, your lung function problems may not improve after quitting, but the latest research studies are starting to show that you may considerably slow the rate at which your lungs disintegrate. As an ex-smoker you'll enjoy fewer days in bed, and your long-suffering spouse won't hear you complaining as much about your feeling lousy. When you quit you will also escape the smoker's constant companions, bronchitis and pneumonia.

It is clear that many smokers ultimately pay a high price for the pleasure of consuming nicotine, but those smokers who don't want their health permanently impaired may be able to quit smoking in time to avoid being another statistic. Even though some profound damage has probably taken place from years of smoking, you can take comfort in the fact that, if given the chance, the body is a self-repairing mechanism.

The Good News On Weight Gain and Your Efforts to Quit Smoking

Perhaps you are finally convinced that quitting is the ticket to longevity, but you still have one thing weighing heavily on your mind — your stomach, hips, and thighs. For many people, especially women, one of the big drawbacks to quitting smoking is weight gain. This is not a trivial issue. When fears of weight gain are placed on top of the mental and physical stress of trying to quit, a powerful set of hurdles stands in your way.

The difference in weight between smokers and nonsmokers is significant but not extreme. Smokers on average weigh from six to ten pounds less than nonsmokers. When a smoker quits, the typical weight gain occurs during the first year and may average over ten pounds. Even in smokers who have not suffered the other withdrawal problems detailed in Chapter Five, concern over added pounds may trigger a relapse.

Why do smokers gain weight when they quit? The relationship between smoking and weight is complex. One of the elements involves an inhibition of hunger which is more in the brain than the stomach. There are several fairly straightforward observations that may help you understand this weighty issue.

Smokers who quit generally start eating more. This should not be thought of as simply compensating for lost "oral gratification." Former smokers have better appetites, in part because the taste buds in the mouth bounce back from the smoke attack and start sending signals to the brain again. Taste buds specializing in sugar sensations are really energized, resulting in diets with generally higher calorie counts.

Nicotine has been proven to play a major role in maintaining reduced weight during smoking. Studies have shown that nicotine may act as an appetite suppressant, leading, most notably, to reduced consumption of sweeter, high-calorie foods, but nicotine also affects the body's general metabolism. It may elevate the baseline rate of energy consumption, which may affect how body fat is metabolized.

As we get older, all of us unfortunately have a hidden regulator that determines our body's weight set point, given our general build, our lifestyle, and the genes we've inherited from our parents. I say "unfortunately" because for many of us the regulator is adjusted a few pounds too high, and we end up riding the roller coaster of weight control. Though we haven't figured out just why, some mechanism in nicotine may also lower the body's weight set point.

If nicotine is important in maintaining a lower body weight in smokers, then it is logical to conclude that nicotine substitution, rather than abstinence, will prevent the weight gain that people who quit smoking normally experience. In fact, many studies have clearly demonstrated that using nicotine gum does decrease the weight gain associated with quitting. The more gum that is consumed, the less the weight gain. These effects have been proven even for long term nicotine gum chewers.

Smokeless tobacco does not alter the sensitivity of taste buds like smoking does. Therefore, when you switch to smokeless tobacco you may find that food immediately starts tasting better. The fact that nicotine replacement reduces the weight gain associated with smoking cessation is also a great reason for choosing the smokeless tobacco solution. Because the average nicotine levels achieved with smokeless tobacco use are very similar to those from smoking, it is possible that you will not experience a big weight gain.

Why Prescription Nicotine Substitutes and Other Quit-Smoking Products and Programs Often Fail

The first thing to reiterate here is that nicotine is absolutely addictive, no matter how the tobacco industry touts the 40 million Americans who have managed to quit. The 40 million figure represents 2.5 percent of all smokers, many of whom may have quit and relapsed several times over a 25 year period.

Don't think I am only talking about veteran smokers who are middle aged or older. A Gallup poll shows that 70 percent of all younger smokers regret that they ever started. Nonetheless, a solid 50 percent of these younger smokers who try to quit cannot, according to Dr. Herbert D. Kleber of the Center on Addiction and Substance Abuse and Dr. David Conney of Columbia University's College of Physicians and Surgeons.

Are you thinking about quitting by gradually reducing the number of cigarettes you smoke each day until you get to zero? Well, think again. This is a tough way to go, with almost no chance of success. In Chapter Five I talked about the reaction of smokers to limitations in cigarette numbers or low nicotine brands. Reducing your daily smokes from 40 to 15 may only be an elaborate illusion with regard to any health benefits.

You can see that millions of Americans are just *not going to quit smoking* no matter what the health professionals say to intimidate them and no matter how much they are harassed by antismoking legislation and/or sin taxes. If you need nicotine, especially after reading Chapter Five, at least get it more safely. While such a "nicotine maintenance program" does not make quitting nicotine use much easier, it also doesn't make quitting nicotine use the major goal. I am primarily concerned with damage control for the smoking epidemic, rather than yet another futile attempt to crush the epidemic in one fell swoop.

The Facts About Non-Tobacco Nicotine Products

Of course, substituting a non-tobacco nicotine alternative or some other drug that simulates nicotine sounds ideal. It would appear to be a great deal more desirable than my lesser-of-two-evils smokeless tobacco thesis. Rather than ignoring such alternatives, I want to discuss these with you and explain why, unfortunately, these strategies are so limited and so often unsuccessful.

You may have heard that nicotine can be provided to the bloodstream of the addicted smoker in the form of chewing gum or by wearing a timed-release skin patch. Often when my program of smokeless tobacco substitution for cigarette smoking is discussed, somebody asks how it is different from the gum or the patch alternative. Actually, I applaud the use of these or any products that may help someone to stop smoking. Once you know the pros and cons associated with them, they may be very useful to you. Here are some facts which may help you decide.

Currently, nicotine substitution products are available only through a prescription from a physician or dentist. Their express purpose is to provide temporary relief from the physical withdrawal symptoms of stopping smoking.

Nicotine Gum

Nicotine chewing gum can be used any time you want a cigarette. When you are given the prescription, your doctor should advise you to chew one piece of gum at a time, up to a maximum of

30 pieces a day. (The manufacturer states that most people will find that ten to twelve pieces per day will be sufficient.) To get the nicotine into your system, it is essential to follow specific chewing instructions. Too many prescriptions are wasted because the gum is not chewed correctly.

The gum should be placed in your mouth, then chewed about fifteen times until a peppery taste or tingling sensation is felt. It should then be "parked" in the cheek area, much like smokeless tobacco, until the taste or tingling is gone (about one minute). The chewing and parking steps should be continued for about 30 minutes, during which time you will absorb the nicotine into your system through the lining of your mouth. Nicotine is not absorbed through the stomach, so swallowing saliva is not the objective.

The gum appears to be safe, but there are some side effects that you should discuss with your doctor or pharmacist. The most obvious advantage of the gum is that it delivers only nicotine to your system, without any of the other substances found in tobacco. However, there are several disadvantages:

1. As I mentioned before, specific chewing instructions must be strictly followed. Even a motivated smoke-quitter can get frustrated by the attention required to properly use the gum.

2. Heavy smokers must often use many pieces of nicotine gum to eliminate the desire for a cigarette — and even after many pieces, they do not get the same nicotine jolt obtained by smoking. The reason: the amount of nicotine in each piece of the gum is low, and it takes 20 to 30 minutes of very careful chewing to achieve optimal release.

3. As with many prescription drugs, the gum does not offer a cost advantage compared to cigarettes. For example, depending on the cigarette brand, a two-pack-a-day smoker spends $120 or less a month. Smokers who need to chew sixteen pieces of gum a day can spend as much as $150 a month at current prices. This discourages many smokers from using chewing gum as a substitute.

4. While it is more socially acceptable to chew gum than to smoke at many job sites or social occasions, one still runs the risk of looking like a ruminant cow or a hyperactive adolescent. Today's compact pouches of smokeless tobacco are more discreet, not to say less tiring, than continuously chewing 10, 20, or 30 pieces of gum per day.

Nicotine Patch

The nicotine patch supplies a constant dose of nicotine through the skin over an 18 or 24 hour period. It is available in three doses which are intended to wean you off nicotine entirely. The main objective of the patch is to supply enough nicotine to reduce withdrawal symptoms without the bother of repeatedly chewing gum. For too many smokers, however, the patch does not supply enough nicotine to prevent craving a cigarette. These individuals are tempted to smoke while the patch is on. Don't! This can be extremely dangerous. The combined nicotine doses can lead to acute heart and circulatory problems. [Author's note: That was the accepted medical wisdom in 1995; however, later studies showed that use of multiple nicotine products did not confer high risk.]

Both of these products are designed to be used only temporarily. The gum is not intended to be used longer than six months, although it is not unusual for people to use the gum much longer. The patch is supposed to be worn for up to four months, but, as seen below, it is not effective as an aid to quitting when it is used longer than six to eight weeks. Also keep in mind that these products are most effective when combined with a formal and comprehensive quit-smoking program that includes emotional and psychological support.

The nicotine patch has failed to help some 75 percent of those who have tried this method of quitting smoking. This means that the patch fails to help three of the four million people that try it each year. On the bright side, it has helped 25 percent of the attempted quitters. Dr. Michael C. Fiore, director of the Center for Tobacco Research and Intervention at the University of Wisconsin, led a team of researchers who reviewed the results of seventeen different studies involving over 5,000 smokers. In this, the most thorough analysis of the nicotine patch ever done, the smoking habits of patch users and dummy patch users were compared to see if the patches were merely functioning as placebos.

The patch does have some physical benefit, and is not merely a psychological aid. One-fourth of the real patch users were still not smoking six months later, while only one-tenth of the phoney patch users were beating their cigarette addiction. Again, we can see that it takes a highly motivated quitter to successfully use the patch. After all, some quitters who did not get any nicotine in their system at all managed to quit. Dr. Fiore also felt that the recommended ten to eighteen weeks on the patch, costing some $350, was too expensive and time-consuming. Many of the successful quitters, he feels, were just as likely to quit after only six to eight weeks. While patch users were advised to take counseling at the same time, Dr. Fiore felt that it made little difference.

Many experts don't think of the nicotine patch as unnecessary or unsuccessful. Dr. Richard D. Hurt, head of the nicotine dependence center at the Mayo Clinic in Rochester, Minnesota, described the patch as "so much better than any other stop-smoking aid." Dr. Hurt conceded that the patch was no miracle cure, as "nicotine dependence is a very complicated disorder."

Darn right it is, and that is why the patch should be considered the best quit-nicotine strategy, but not necessarily the best quit-smoking one. Smokeless tobacco is overlooked as another effective quit-smoking concept. This is because of a stubborn insistence on an all-or-nothing approach to fighting tobacco when the primary target should be smoking. The average smoker, especially one who has tried and failed to quit, will be reluctant to invest in the time, patience, and expense of either of the prescription nicotine delivery systems. The short-term, more physically satisfying solution that will save more lives sooner remains smokeless tobacco.

Low Tar and Low Nicotine Cigarettes

You may have already tried this first step to quitting or to reduce your risks of medical problems including premature death or cancer or heart disease, but you likely accomplished neither, which is why it is on the bottom of my list of solutions. Smoking is the problem — not the nicotine (as established in Chapter Five) — so downgrading from Camel to True may actually make you a less happy smoker because of lower nicotine levels, and you will probably have no less risk of serious lung and heart diseases.

The sole purpose of these cigarettes is to ostensibly provide you with lower doses of tar and nicotine, but even this objective is in serious jeopardy. The Federal Trade Commission and other sources have cast doubts on the contents of low tar and nicotine cigarettes. While smokers feel they are using a less hazardous product, tests show that smokers subconsciously take deeper drags on these cigarettes to get the equivalent amount of nicotine out of them.

Instead of reduced tar, the smoker of the "safe" cigarette is likely taking in as much if not more tar than ever.

The advertised lower amounts of tar and nicotine are based on machines that take two-second puffs once every minute. But you aren't a machine. You want the nicotine and will therefore take more and deeper puffs from these cigarettes to satisfy that need. Scientists monitoring the nicotine level in the blood of smokers often cannot tell which smokers use full-flavored cigarettes and which smoke the so-called low nicotine cigarettes. Sadly, these products don't make you a healthier smoker, only a harder working one.

Unlike smokeless tobacco, in which more consistent nicotine levels are available essentially without effort (see Chapter Seven), the amount of nicotine recovered from a cigarette depends as much on the smoker as on the cigarette. These "light" cigarettes may do more harm than good. More frequent and stronger puffing means more nicotine, and more tar as well. While the tiny holes in the filter paper of these cigarettes do make a difference in the substances recorded by cigarette machines, they make no difference in your lungs and bloodstream when you drag harder on that pack of Trues rather than mildly puffing on that half pack of Camels. From a standpoint of cigarette tobacco, what would make better sense? Instead of reducing the nicotine content of tobacco, why not make a cigarette with more nicotine, so that the smoker 's needs are met with a minimum of puffing. Well, tune in to this.

The (Wh)Y-1 Debate

The congressional hearings, which I have referred to several times in this book, have become more and more curious. Dr. David Kessler, Commissioner of the Food and Drug Administration, told a Congressional hearing on June 21, 1994 that a major cigarette company produced a strain of tobacco with twice the nicotine of other plants. Brown & Williamson Tobacco Corporation, makers of Viceroy, Richland and Raleigh brands, at first denied that it secretly developed this genetically engineered tobacco in Brazil. After being confronted with evidence, however, the company admitted to having at least three million pounds of the specially developed tobacco, called Y-1, in its American warehouses.

95

Y-1 was developed from a 1970's experiment by the United States Department of Agriculture. With genetic alterations, a tobacco plant was produced which contained 6.2 percent nicotine by weight instead of the normal 3 percent in naturally-cured tobacco.

Let's say that for every unit of nicotine you need as a smoker, you also absorb a unit of tar, for a one to one ratio. Lowering the tar exposure — let's say by one-half — through some method of filtration also lowers the nicotine proportionately, making you work twice as hard. However, if the nicotine to tar ratio is increased to two to one, you will now get your one unit of nicotine for exactly one half the tar.

Dr. Kessler felt that the tobacco companies were tinkering with cigarette ingredients in an attempt to control their customers' "nicotine addiction." He was using this premise to move the FDA closer to the regulation of tobacco as a drug, which many fear is just the first step toward prohibition.

Y-1 is important to this book because it illustrates that cigarette companies have recognized the problem with their delivery system and that they have gone to great lengths to try to deliver nicotine to smokers while reducing their exposure to the harmful by-products of tobacco combustion. It also demonstrates that tobacco control specialists are stepping up their efforts toward tobacco's ultimate regulation and prohibition. Representative Henry A. Waxman (D-California) got it right when he called cigarettes "chemistry sets in a tube." If the smoker has to get nicotine, let it be without combustion and without the "599 chemical additives" like ammonium hydroxide. Let's get the debate back on track by focusing on the need for a better, safer nicotine delivery system — smokeless tobacco.

Other Quit-Smoking Programs

Don't mistake my pragmatism for defeatism. Millions of people have successfully quit all tobacco products, and you should try to be one of them. This book does not contest the fact that the best (although not by any means the only) option for you is to quit tobacco use altogether.

With this in mind, I include the more traditional quit-smoking programs and advice listed below. As my program has already been attacked by most of these organizations, you might have expected me to react by not including these options and not mentioning these agencies, or I might have listed them in the back of the book in unreadable "micro" print. However, that would be defeating the broader goal of reducing the nation's death toll from tobacco use. Thus, I return the harsh (and unfair) criticism of my program with unqualified support of the following:

Your Dentist or Physician

Your dentist or physician can serve as a first contact for information available from the agencies or groups listed below. Many doctors provide educational materials, advice, encouragement and even nicotine substitution. The American Dental Association and the American Medical Association provide extensive supportive literature which is often at the doctor's office for the asking.

But don't hesitate to ask your doctor about my program. Opposition to the smokeless tobacco solution from the medical establishment does not guarantee a negative judgement from the nation's individual practicing physicians, researchers, health educators, and scientists. These individuals are far more willing to form an opinion only after carefully weighing the evidence, which is a far cry from the knee-jerk reaction on the part of many organizations.

American Cancer Society

This organization supports quit-smoking programs in local communities throughout the nation. Volunteers conduct quit-smoking programs, and the group produces numerous self-help publications.

American Lung Association

Self-help literature and videos are available from this organization. Your spouse or friend may have showed you these shock videos in an attempt to scare you out of smoking.

Lung Health Centers

In larger medical centers and hospitals, federally funded lung health centers provide a spectrum of programs, often targeted to individuals with common interests, goals or specific needs. They combine quit-smoking programs with behavioral and clinical medical research.

In conclusion, if you are determined to stop smoking — and your nicotine addiction — then the instructional materials listed in this chapter may be appropriate for you. But the key is the nicotine, which you must be committed to giving up altogether. This is an admirable goal, but many smokers may find it impossible to achieve.

Throughout your smoky career, you may have tried many or all of these alternatives. Polls indicate that 75 percent of all smokers want to quit. In any year, over one-third make it for a day, and 28 percent throw the cancer sticks away for at least a week. However, because of nicotine addiction's long reach, even many months or years after the last cigarette is smoked, most attempts at quitting are ultimately unsuccessful. In any year, less than 10 percent of smokers who try to quit do so successfully. Formal quit-smoking programs have been in existence since 1955 and have become sophisticated and complex, but relapse rates remain high.

If you are one of the millions who cannot stay away from cigarettes without debilitating discomfort, you owe it to yourself to try taking in the same nicotine with an alternative form of tobacco enjoyment. The idea of switching to smokeless tobacco might make more sense now, so let's take a detailed look at the smokeless tobacco solution.

~ ~ ~

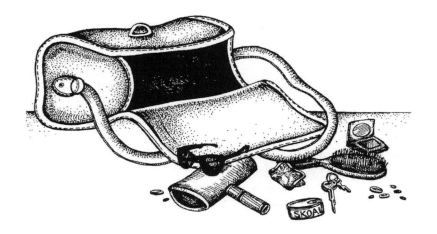

Chapter Seven
The Smokeless Tobacco Solution

Chapter Seven
The Smokeless Tobacco Solution

skoal \ skol \ n [Danish skaal, lit., cup]:
a toast to someone's health, well-being or prosperity.
— Webster's Third New International Dictionary

By now I am sure you understand your physical need, as a cigarette smoker, for nicotine. Smoking is a very efficient way to get nicotine into your system. By inhaling smoke, you speed nicotine to your brain in seconds.

However, nicotine is only one of about 3,000 chemicals that your body absorbs when smoking a cigarette. Some of these are responsible for the high rates of lung and airway cancers, heart attacks, strokes, and emphysema detailed in Chapter Three.

Is there another efficient way to absorb the same amount of nicotine without as many side effects? The answer is yes. A quick, longer-lasting nicotine high is available from products that are widely available without prescription and far safer than cigarettes. These products are collectively called smokeless tobacco.

With everything this book is saying about choosing smokeless tobacco over cigarettes, I hope you aren't alarmed when I say that smokeless tobacco, especially moist snuff, may have a higher concentration of nicotine than cigarettes. This is not a cause for alarm for two reasons. First, nicotine is not the cause of widespread disease and death in smokers — as you have discovered in Chapter Five. Second, regardless of the tobacco used, the amount of nicotine available on average to smokers and smokeless tobacco users is remarkably similar at 150 to 200 milligrams a day.

Comparing Nicotine in Cigarettes and Smokeless Tobacco

The nicotine content of cigarettes ranges from 1.5 percent to 2.5 percent by weight, according to figures in many published studies. For you to be convinced to try smokeless tobacco, you'll need some immediate physical satisfaction in order not to fight the switch.

In order to have the best information available for this solution, my University of Alabama at Birmingham-based research group determined the nicotine level of eleven top brands of smokeless tobacco. The concentration varies according to factors like moisture content, additives, and the varieties of the tobacco itself.

You might have seen the chart below, as our study was widely cited in reporting the nicotine content of smokeless tobacco by specific brand for the first time. The chart might also guide you, the tobacco-switcher, in deciding which product is best for you. Although for completeness we evaluated brands of loose leaf and plug tobacco, you will almost surely want to start out with moist snuff, as I explain in more detail later in the chapter.

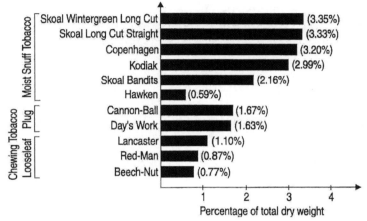

Nicotine Levels in Eleven Top Brands of Smokeless Tobacco Products

You can now easily understand how the concentration of nicotine in smokeless tobacco products might result in blood nicotine levels as high and almost as quickly achieved as cigarette smoking. However, as a smoker you want more than a chart full of numbers; you want that tobacco pleasure. Well, go ahead and try some smokeless tobacco. You'll see in minutes that the medical advice in this book is not aimed at reducing your pleasure nor that familiar nicotine buzz that gets you through your day, but is aimed instead at eliminating your smoke, your guilt, and the impending pain in your vital organs and bank account.

The use of smokeless tobacco is associated with far fewer and less serious health effects than smoking. Best of all, contrary to popular opinion, smokeless tobacco can be used almost invisibly. The dramatics and crudity of the typical major league baseball player shooting out his saliva has nothing to do with the sanitary and polite ways to satisfy a nicotine craving with a small pouch of snuff tobacco. There will be more on the mechanics of using smokeless tobacco products later.

This section of the book provides you with much of the positive information you will need to ease your painless transition from cigarette smoking to smokeless tobacco. You've already gotten enough negatives from your family, the media, and the first six chapters of this book. This is where I fine tune the indiscriminate attack on tobacco. The lifesaving switch to snuff can become a matter of urgent public health policy if sober analysis replaces hysteria. The current mantra against smokeless tobacco is one that dismisses these high nicotine products as unacceptably serious health hazards.

Exploding the Myths About Smokeless Tobacco

Let me destroy the myth that smokeless tobacco is as dangerous as smoking. To accomplish this goal I will present concrete statistics, something that is never done in the war being waged against smokeless tobacco products. Without guilt or fear, you will soon be able, with the smokeless tobacco product best suited to your taste, lifestyle, and needs, to join the many smokeless tobacco users who gave up cigarettes to live happily ever after (or at least as long as people usually live).

The Health Concerns of Smokeless Tobacco Use

You are probably still thinking of everything negative you have heard all these years about smokeless tobacco and oral cancer, and you are now ready to ask, "Isn't smokeless tobacco at least half as dangerous as cigarette smoking?" The answer is a resounding *no*! In their zeal to convince the American public that tobacco is inherently evil, the antitobacco zealots (discussed more thoroughly in Chapter Eight) have created the illusion that all forms of tobacco produce the same health problems.

The misinformation comes from the highest sources, so you can't be blamed for your misperceptions. In 1992, the Surgeon General warned of the potential for an "epidemic" of oral cancer related to smokeless tobacco use. This unfortunate misconception is so deeply ingrained that even many physicians do not really understand how much safer smokeless tobacco is. Let's examine the facts and the real numbers behind the antitobacco frenzy.

Smokeless tobacco use can lead to some observable health problems. The primary concern is the increased risk of oral cancer. The best research conducted so far was published in the prestigious *New England Journal Medicine* in 1981 and has been cited in the cancer research literature over 200 times.

Oral cancer occurs rarely in people who don't use tobacco products. The rate is about 6 cases per 100,000 people each year. The 1981 study concluded that the annual rate of oral cancer in long-term smokeless tobacco users is about four times the nonuser rate, or 26 cases per 100,000. That is, for every 100,000 people who have used smokeless tobacco for a long time, 26 individuals develop oral cancer each year. [Author's note: Information released after this book was written documented that this study only applied to dry powdered snuff, an uncommon smokeless product used mainly by women in the Southern U.S. Moist snuff and chewing tobacco use have far lower risks. For more information, see http://rodutobaccotruth.blogspot.com/2010/04/three-decades-of-smokeless-tobacco.html]

You might hear some antitobacco crusaders say that the oral cancer risk for smokeless tobacco users is a much more impressive 50. But this is only for cancer of the gum, a very rare cancer. The rate of gum cancer in nonusers of tobacco is a minuscule one-half of a case per 100,000 people annually. Even if you multiply by 50, the number of cases due to smokeless tobacco use is still only 26 per 100,000.

What does this mean in real terms? Let's take the 46 million smokers as an example. If all smokers were instead addicted to smokeless tobacco, only 12,000 new cases of oral cancer (with a 50 percent survival rate) could be expected each year. This is only one twentieth of all cancers that now result from smoking, and one tenth of smoking related lung cancer cases! I haven't even mentioned the reduction in heart disease and emphysema deaths yet. *If all 46 million smokers used smokeless tobacco instead, the United States would see, at worst, 6,000 deaths from oral cancer, versus the current 419,000 deaths from smoking-related cancers, heart problems, and lung disease.*

If you think of all the lives and millions of health dollars that could be saved, you will appreciate how crucial the message of this book is. Of course, you may still look at the statistics and say that smokeless tobacco is still a contributing cause of oral cancer. But full implementation of my program would result in only one-half the number of mouth cancer cases currently attributed to smoking. You could more easily say that the smokeless tobacco solution, other than everyone quitting smoking, can be the greatest single factor in the battle to eradicate oral cancer.

You don't have to be an Einstein to understand relativity. Relative to cigarettes, smokeless tobacco products are a godsend. Don't get me wrong, I am not casually suggesting a switch from lung cancer to oral cancer, which is the theme song of some of my critics. But I can't resist mentioning a major difference between these cancers. Oral cancer is easily detected in its earlier stages; while lung cancer is very difficult to diagnose before it has spread throughout the body. This accounts for the far higher five-year survival rate for oral cancers (48 percent) than for those deeply hidden in the lung (12 percent).

How likely is the Surgeon General's predicted oral cancer "epidemic" among smokeless tobacco users? Let's look at America's most observable long-term users. Almost 25 percent of men over sixteen years of age in West Virginia use smokeless tobacco, a pattern which has been established for decades and is considerably above the national average of 6 percent. Contrary to the beliefs of the tobacco-bashers, a smaller percentage of these West Virginians died from oral cancer from 1950 to 1980 than in the United States as a whole. So much for our government's oral cancer epidemic scare.

You may be convinced by now that smokeless tobacco use is far healthier than cigarettes, but I still might be accused of being a pick-your-poison promoter. Let me again turn to some critical research conducted here at the University of Alabama at Birmingham.

How Smokeless Tobacco Will Add 7.8 Years to Your Life

I conducted the following study under the guidance and with the assistance of Dr. Philip Cole, a professor of epidemiology here at UAB. We had a very simple goal, to estimate the life expectancy of 35-year-old American men who smoke cigarettes, use smokeless tobacco, and don't use tobacco products at all.

For nonusers and smokers, we used death rate statistics from the American Cancer Society. These statistics came from studies of smoking and death rates among more than 1 million Americans aged 30 or older.

For smokeless tobacco dippers and chewers we used standard methods to determine the risk for oral cancer. To make sure we didn't underestimate the risk of oral cancer, we doubled the best current estimate. This allowed us to compare the deaths due to oral cancer in smokeless tobacco users with the deaths in smokers and nonusers.

The results of our analysis, translated into projected years of life, reveal that the average remaining life expectancy of a 35-year-old smokeless tobacco user is 45.92 years, which is merely four-hundredths of a year less than the nonuser of tobacco. Statistically speaking, use of full-bodied tobacco products with all the nicotine of cigarettes will cost the smokeless tobacco user only fifteen days of life! That's about 2,780 more days than the cigarette smoker lives.

Now, this figure of fifteen days is a sharp contrast to the minimum seven and eight-tenths years of average life expectancy you lose by being a smoker. Both the 35-year-old tobacco abstainer and the smokeless tobacco user will live on average to be 80.9 years of age, compared to your expected departure at only 73.1 years of age. Only 67 percent of smokers will be alive at age 70, compared with over 87 percent of smokeless tobacco users and nonusers of tobacco. That's not to say that it's too late even for a 70-year-old to benefit by switching to snuff, but the younger a smoker is when he or she converts, the more gain (in life expectancy) and the less pain.

If anything, we likely overestimated the health impact of smokeless tobacco use because we applied the oral cancer risk equally at all ages after 35 years. In actuality, when oral cancer occurs in long term snuff users, they are generally over the age of 70. In one of the largest studies of its kind, the rare smokeless tobacco users who developed oral cancer averaged 78 years of age and had used smokeless tobacco for about 55 years.

How Swede It Is

When studying oral cancer and its impact on society, it's tough to ignore Sweden. Swedish per capita consumption of moist snuff has been the highest in the world *for the entire century*. In 1920, when use in America was also near its height, Sweden consumed a whopping three and six-tenths pounds of smokeless tobacco for every citizen over fifteen years old. And Swedes still consumed a pound of smokeless tobacco per person in the 1970's. This is far from being indicative of a backward or old fashioned country; Sweden's standard of living is among the highest in the world.

Besides highly developed cultural and social amenities, the country also boasts a high life expectancy. Surely, if smokeless tobacco posed significant health problems this would not be so.

The Swedes have had many years to study the effects of smokeless tobacco use. One would imagine Stockholm to be the oral cancer capital of the world, but this is absolutely not the case. In fact, Sweden has one of the lowest rates of oral cancer in Europe and is below that of the United States (where only 4 percent of the population uses smokeless tobacco products with any regularity). Apparently, all that dipping and snuffing has not cost the Swedes a high rate of oral cancer at all. Why not? Because smoking rates in Sweden have been relatively low.

While many Swedes were taking their tobacco pleasure without burning it and inhaling the fumes, they were avoiding the higher lung cancer rates plaguing countries all around them that have higher smoking rates. This is the kind of common sense solution I want to see used by smokers in the United States — and everywhere else where one hears the sound of lighting a match followed by that familiar hacking cough. Tragically, American movies and marketing have had international reach in their portrayal of cigarettes as the magical purveyors of celebrity vapors and cool nonchalance. Worldwide cancer and cardiovascular statistics are not where America's legacy should be most evident.

Can smokeless tobacco be lumped together with cigarettes when examining heart disease? I reviewed the evidence in detail in Chapter Three, and the answer is definitely not.

Smokeless tobacco use, like cigarette smoking, can cause some minor problems involving the gums, and any tobacco use (including smoking) can stain teeth, dentures, and fillings. Of course, compared with the list of serious illnesses associated with smoking, these are trivial problems that can be easily monitored and managed by your dentist. If switching to snuff prompts you to see a dentist twice a year, your teeth and your entire mouth will be better off.

White Patches

Using smokeless tobacco over long periods of time will have some effect on the lining of the mouth where the pinch or pouch of tobacco is placed. Over time this small area will get slightly thicker; it might even turn white. This is not unusual at all for a frequent smokeless tobacco user and is comparable to a tennis player developing calluses where he or she grips the racket. Using pouches of snuff delays the appearance of the white patch, but eventually 40 percent to 60 percent of smokeless tobacco users will develop what researchers call "leukoplakia" (literally, *leuko* meaning white and *plakia* meaning plaque or patch). While the official medical name for this white patch of skin sounds ominous, studies have shown over and over that these calluses hardly ever turn into something more serious. Occasionally changing the placement of your pinch or pouch can also keep white patch development at a minimum.

Despite research to the contrary, antitobacco troopers have been very aggressive in trying to link this white patch to oral cancer. As an oral pathologist, I have researched this issue very carefully As documented above, the risk of oral cancer among smokeless tobacco users — including those with the white patches of skin on the lining of their cheek — is very small. When compared to the risk of oral cancer among smokers, it is almost criminal to implicate smokeless tobacco as the bigger problem when it is clearly the single workable solution.

While leukoplakia has been associated with smokeless tobacco use, it also occurs among cigarette smokers. These white patches are a far greater concern among smokers because they are much more likely eventually to develop into oral cancer. When you switch to smokeless tobacco you drastically reduce your risk of oral cancer. This fact needs to be written large because too many of my colleagues are subject to the propaganda campaign against all tobacco products, and they share the popular misconception that smokeless tobacco is somehow associated with a higher risk of oral cancer than cigarettes.

This chapter and this book are necessary to counter published statements that are not always scientifically objective and accurate. By leaving no medical stone unturned and providing you with verifiable information, I want to encourage you to take the steps you need to adopt a healthier lifestyle. In offering you the smokeless tobacco solution that my purist colleagues prefer to suppress, I am maintaining rigorous scientific standards in presenting research on tobacco use and nicotine addiction. My research has a practical and realistic side, and it is the best way to save thousands of lives right away.

The white patches and any other minor problems related to smokeless tobacco use are quite visible and detectable by the average user. Regular and thorough checkups by your dentist and dental hygienist will detect any possible problems early enough for effective treatment. Unlike the many deadly and insidious health dangers of smoking, smokeless tobacco can only affect areas of your mouth that are easily examined.

The Warnings On Smokeless Tobacco Products

No matter how reassured you might be that the can of snuff you are going to purchase is the healthiest way to stay with tobacco, you might get a bit disconcerted when you read the government-mandated warnings on the side of the container. The three rotating warnings printed on the round, flat cans of snuff are purposely vague, but they might shake up the smoke-quitter who was looking forward to enjoying some tobacco pleasure without facing serious death threats. Let's look at these three warnings and comment on their scientific truth:

1. Warning: This product may cause gum disease and tooth loss.
2. Warning: This product may cause mouth cancer.
3. Warning: This product is not a safe alternative to cigarettes.

Warning number one is only valid in that smokeless tobacco might slightly increase your chances of damaging the gum or teeth. With the regular checkups I have already recommended, any such gum damage would be caught too early to pose a serious problem. More importantly, candy and other sugar-laden snack foods are better established threats to teeth and gums, yet no such warning is printed on the packages of those products.

The second warning is more ominous because it contains the "C word," cancer, but now you can evaluate its true meaning. The antismoking crusaders have swung their maces at everything containing tobacco or nicotine in their well-meaning war on cigarettes. They have thrown around the word "cancer" to trash smokeless tobacco as a "major cause of oral cancer" without even looking at the statistics in a meaningful way. It is like condemning pedestrians as a leading cause of traffic accidents.

The third warning is simply ludicrous. Are automobiles safe? How about lawnmowers, boats, aspirin, red meat, and raw oysters? By applying the absolute definition of "safe," nothing measures up. In fact, if the smoke bashers, the media, and my colleagues in the medical profession can muster an ounce of sympathy for the hooked smoker, they will also look beyond the tobacco witch hunt and hail smokeless tobacco as a realistic solution for smokers who cannot or will not quit.

While the information above will help smokers add years of life by switching to these smokeless tobacco products, some critics raised the possibility that our data will influence the debate over the tobacco industry's motives for promoting smokeless tobacco products. (For an example, see the *New York Daily News* of May 5, 1994.) They charge that young people hooked on nicotine from smokeless tobacco will move on to cigarettes.

It is clear from our data above that smokeless tobacco has the nicotine potency to create new addicts in addition to serving as the safer alternative for someone hooked on more dangerous cigarettes. Just as it is unlikely that teenagers will read our study before deciding what unacceptable behavior is "cool," it would be bizarre for anyone to interpret our work as a defense of the tobacco industry whose cigarettes I am constantly indicting here. Switching from smokeless tobacco to cigarettes, instead of vice versa, is the very antithesis of this book's intent.

It is tragic that smokeless tobacco use has increased among adolescent American boys, often as a result of their emulating baseball players with their wads of chewing tobacco. The increase in smokeless tobacco use among older teens between 1970 and 1985 has been estimated on the low end at 36 percent by the *British Journal of Addiction* to an incredible high of 300 percent by the United States Department of Education. The Centers for Disease Control in Atlanta reports that one in five adolescent male students are at least occasional users of smokeless tobacco. I don't want to see anyone but older, hardened, long-term smokers turning to these products as the safer delivery system for their nicotine addiction; for these very people, these products are a wise choice.

From Theory to Reality

I am aware that even six chapters of persuasion won't necessarily move you to put tobacco in your mouth. It's my job now to move you from the theoretical realm of statistics to the practical sphere of action. Putting that first small pouch of flavored tobacco between your cheek and gum will seem much more natural once you read about the various tobacco products.

The Return to Smokeless Tobacco Starts Now

In Chapter Two, I explained how cigarettes became synonymous with tobacco use earlier in the century. All the antismoking measures and proclamations don't differentiate between cigarettes and other tobacco products because smokeless tobacco use is essentially nonexistent in the big cities. If snuff can make a temporary comeback, it will give current cigarette smokers a chance to catch their breath.

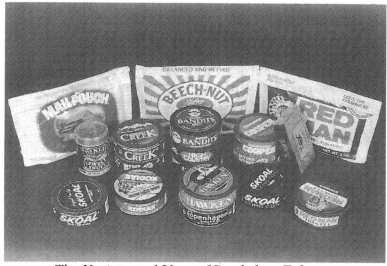

The Variety and Uses of Smokeless Tobacco

The Variety and Uses of Smokeless Tobacco

For you adult readers who are ready to try the switch, you will see many smokeless tobacco products in your local supermarket or convenience store. Hundreds of products are sold throughout the country, although a far more limited selection of brands will be available in any one region. The bewildering number and variety of choices may be classified into three categories: dry powdered snuff, loose leaf and plug chewing tobacco, and moist snuff. Although I will concentrate on products in the last category, you should be familiar with the other types.

Dry Powdered Snuff

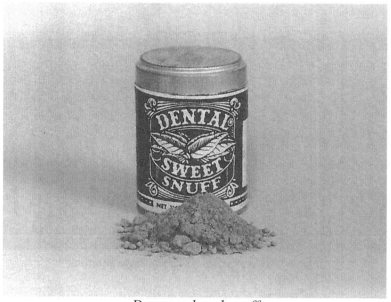

Dry powdered snuff

Dry, finely powdered snuff was introduced into Europe in 1559 by Jean Nicot, the French ambassador to Sebastian, King of Portugal. It remained popular in France, England, and Scotland well into the 19th century. This form of tobacco was inhaled through the nose and resulted in both rapid nicotine intake and a vigorous sneeze, which was considered a cleansing and generally pleasant experience. Today it is the least popular form of smokeless tobacco; it is used mainly in the rural southern United States by placing a small amount of powder in the mouth. Sometimes you will see this type of snuff referred to as "sweet" or "Scotch" snuff.

Loose Leaf and Plug Chewing Tobacco

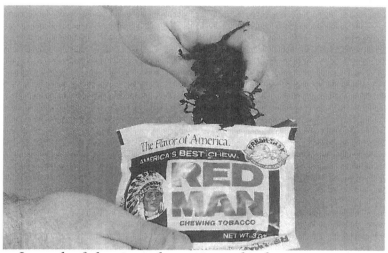

Loose leaf chewing tobacco is used in larger quantities

Loose leaf chewing tobacco consists of shredded tobacco leaves and stems and is packaged in foil pouches. Using Burley tobacco, which absorbs additives, chewing tobacco is also heavily sweetened and flavored. Loose leaf brands include such recognizable names as Mail Pouch and Beech-Nut, as well as more evocative names such as Red Horse and Chattanooga Chew. Appeal to the rough and tough outdoorsman is made in the names Rough Country, Trophy, and Work Horse.

Plug tobacco, an original American form of tobacco, received its name from its method of production. In the mid-1800's, small factories in the Southeast drilled holes in trees such as maple, elm, and poplar which contained a sweet sap. When tobacco was "plugged" into these holes, it absorbed some of the sap and underwent fermentation. After several weeks it was removed, packaged, and sold. That down-on-the-farm feeling is still strong.

You'll see names like Days Work, Cannon-Ball, Bloodhound, and Brown's Mule on these packages.

When smokeless tobacco is mentioned, most Americans immediately and unfortunately think of loose leaf chewing tobacco. This bulky form of tobacco is used in larger quantities than snuff. It forms the typical swollen cheek appearance as it is chewed by professional baseball players. The large cud of tobacco generates a lot of saliva which is generally not swallowed. It is this most blatant use of chewing tobacco, accompanied by continuous long distance spitting, which has given all smokeless tobacco products an undeserved reputation as socially undesirable. Fewer and fewer ballplayers are using this form of tobacco, and those that do are often mixing it with bubble gum.

Moist Snuff

Moist snuff is a hybrid between powdered dry snuff and scrap chewing tobacco. It is ground to the consistency of finely chopped parsley, but remains moist. Although several flavors are now available, moist snuff does not generally contain as much sweetener as chewing tobacco.

Moist snuff is used in small amounts, generally as much as can be grasped between the thumb and forefinger in a "pinch." The tobacco is then placed into the mouth just inside the lower lip between the cheek and gum. Nicotine is absorbed with remarkable speed through the cheek, giving the user a nicotine "buzz" very similar to that achieved by smoking a cigarette. In fact, light cigarette smokers often report a rapid and powerful effect, so the amount of snuff used must be adjusted according to the individual user's needs.

Because moist snuff is finely ground, making it hard to contain in one spot inside the cheek, manufacturers have come up with a system that is much more user friendly. They have packaged pinch-sized portions of snuff in small tea-bag type paper pouches, which can be neatly and quickly placed inside the cheek. The pouches are no larger than a piece of chewing gum or a breath mint, making them virtually invisible to place and use. They also don't disintegrate, which makes the tobacco easy to remove after use. Women, educators, or anyone who cannot smoke, chew, or spit without social consequences can discreetly enjoy moist snuff — even in public.

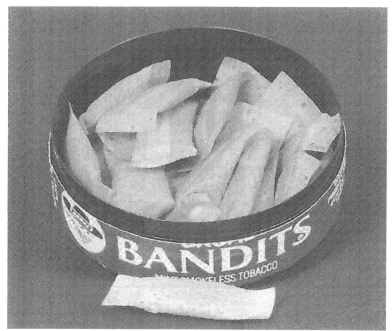

Paper pouches of moist snuff

Moist snuff has many advantages over chewing and plug tobacco. This virtually undetectable form of enjoying tobacco is my primary recommendation for smokers who are switching. I have interviewed many professionals who use moist snuff all the time. It is often in their mouths, undetected, throughout their business and professional activities.

But what about spitting? Does this continue to be an obvious sign of smokeless tobacco use? Not with moist snuff. Because it is used in small quantities, snuff doesn't produce the large amounts of saliva that plague chewing and plug tobacco users. Small amounts of saliva containing tobacco juice can be swallowed without upsetting the stomach. Many of our switchers, including women, find that they do not have to spit any saliva at all. Moist snuff allows you to get your daily nicotine fix without matches, ashtrays, or spittoons.

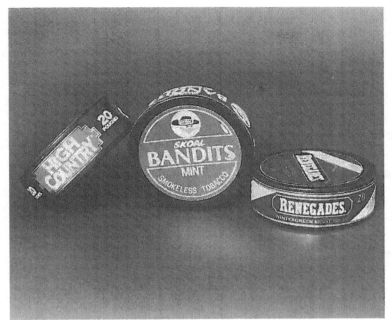

The three brands of moist snuff currently available in pouches

Some stomachs are sensitive, so if you find that you do need to spit, you can discreetly do so in a cup, mug, or empty soft drink can. The casual observer cannot tell whether you are sipping a drink or releasing saliva. You may also find that spitting will only be needed during the first five or ten minutes, when the tobacco juices are most concentrated.

If you find that one prepackaged pouch is not strong enough, try two. They are so small that even using two at a time is not difficult. You may also try the loose form of moist snuff. At first it may take some practice to keep the tobacco from travelling throughout your mouth. Try the long cut products first because they can be packed together more easily during use.

Making the Switch from Smoking to Smokeless Tobacco
How Do You Start?

Go out and buy some smokeless tobacco. You should buy the prepackaged pouches first. Skoal Bandits, made by United States Tobacco, is the most popular brand, but the Pinkerton Tobacco Co.

has recently introduced two new pouches named High Country and Renegades. Bandits are sold in several flavors, including regular and classic tobacco flavors, mint, and wintergreen. Smokers who enjoy menthol cigarettes usually prefer either the wintergreen or mint flavor. Each package contains 20 to 25 individual pouches.

There are many other brands and flavors of moist snuff on the market. In the table are some of the most popular brands that should be widely available.

Brand	Nicotine Level	Flavor	Other Characteristics
Skoal Regular Cut	High	Tobacco	Finely ground
		Wintergreen	
Skoal Long Cut	High	Tobacco	Packs well
		Wintergreen	
		Cherry	
		Spearmint	
		Mint	
		Classic tobacco	
Copenhagen	High	Strong tobacco	Finely ground
Kodiak	High	Strong tobacco	Finely ground
Skoal Bandits	Medium	Regular	Pouches
		Wintergreen	
		Mint	
		Classic	
Hawken	Low	Wintergreen	Packs well
Other moist snuff brands include Redwood, Silver Creek Wintergreen, Gold River Long Cut, Cooper Long Cut Wintergreen, Red Man Long Cut, Garrett, High Country Pouches, Renegades Pouches.			

The table lists many of the moist snuff products available as this book goes to press. In addition, it provides you with some information concerning the variety of flavors, packaging, and nicotine content as indicated by our research.

When Should You Use Smokeless Tobacco, and How?

It is important to establish a new ritual with smokeless tobacco, to replace the old ritual of lighting up a cigarette. It is best to think of each pinch or pouch of moist snuff as replacing a cigarette. Follow these simple and easy directions:

1. Wait until you would normally smoke to use smokeless tobacco.

2. Open up a fresh can, take a pouch, and place it between your lower cheek and gum. I recommend starting with a Bandit.

If you are a moderate smoker (less than one pack of cigarettes a day), allow the Bandit to stay in place only for a few minutes the first time you "unlight" up, until the desire for a cigarette wears off. Don't overdo it. Smokeless tobacco is powerful stuff — that's why it works so easily for so many smokers.

If you are a heavy smoker (one to one-and-a-half packs a day), you'll probably find that a pouch works well. If you are a very heavy smoker (two packs a day or more), try the pouch first, but don't get discouraged if you need to keep it in place longer for that satisfied feeling.

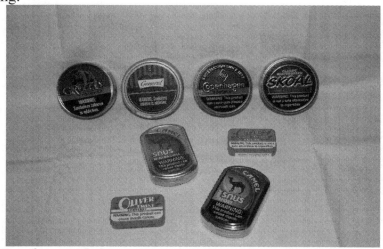

Spit-free smokeless tobacco products in pouches and pellets, available throughout the U.S. in 2013.

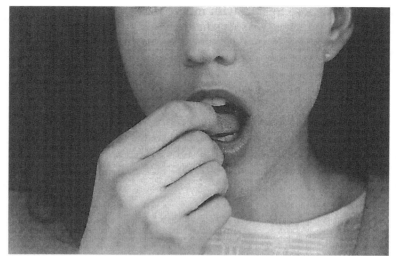

Placing a pouch of moist sniff between the cheek and lower gum

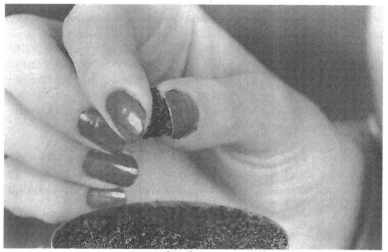

A pinch of moist snuff

3. If you choose to start with moist snuff which isn't prepackaged in pouches, grasp a small amount between your thumb and forefinger. Place this "pinch" of moist snuff between your lower lip and gum near the corner of your mouth or back further in your cheek. With very little practice you should be able to keep the tobacco in place.

I suggest starting with a small pinch, since the loose form of moist snuff will permit more and faster nicotine absorption. Check out the previous table for relative nicotine concentrations in the most popular brands.

How Do You Handle Spitting?

Try smokeless tobacco for the first time in the privacy of your home, where you can spit out any tobacco juices if you feel you need to. With progressive usage, if you find that you need to spit, you can very discreetly use an empty soft drink can or a cup. Friends, colleagues, or family do not have to know whether you are drinking or spitting. Remember, unlike passive smoke, there is no such thing as passive saliva. While you are doing your health a huge favor, you are also eliminating a major cause of conflict and debate — the passive smoking issue. You will be able to enjoy tobacco wherever and whenever you choose — in your office, public buildings, airports, restaurants, and planes — without eliciting stares and harassment from nonusers of tobacco.

As you become accustomed to smokeless tobacco, you may want to test how much to spit and for how long. Many smokeless tobacco users in my program don't spit at all or only spit long enough to eliminate the concentrated juices.

If spitting the concentrated juices for the first couple minutes is a must, use a handkerchief or tissue to dab your lips a few times.

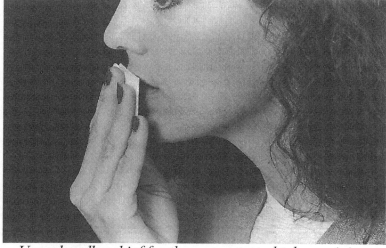

Use a handkerchief for the concentrated tobacco juices

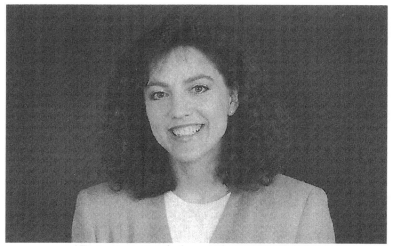

Enjoying smokeless tobacco invisibly

How Will You Know When You've Got the Right Amount?

Properly used, smokeless tobacco should satisfy you within a few minutes. Of course, nothing will speed nicotine to your brain as fast as burning tobacco and inhaling it directly into your lungs. A few minutes after placing a pinch or a pouch of smokeless tobacco, you should feel one of the following:

1. You may feel just about right, indicating that you have achieved the same effects using a pouch or a pinch of smokeless tobacco as smoking a cigarette.

2. You may feel unsatisfied and still want a cigarette. The pouch may not have been strong enough to meet your nicotine needs. Try switching to another brand of pouches, or you may want to try one of the loose moist snuff products. If you are already using the loose form, try a larger pinch or sample a brand with a higher nicotine level.

3. You may get a nicotine buzz accompanied by light-headedness, nausea, flushing, a rapid heartbeat and/or dizziness. You overdid it. I have seen heavy smokers who were amazed by the strength of smokeless tobacco. Next time, reduce the amount of tobacco, switch to a brand that delivers a lower nicotine hit, or take

the smokeless tobacco out sooner. Remember, smoking a cigarette takes only a few minutes. Smokeless tobacco provides the same blood level of nicotine as cigarette smoking, but it takes a little longer. On the other hand, the nicotine level stays higher longer. The advantage of this is that most switchers use less smokeless tobacco to achieve the same effect.

For How Long Should You Use Smokeless Tobacco Each Time?

There is great variation among smokeless tobacco users as to how long to leave the pinch or pouch in place. Some users discard the tobacco within one-half hour, replacing it with fresh tobacco more frequently. Other users find that one dip in the morning may be left in place until lunch, with dips after lunch and dinner offering similar long lasting satisfaction. The longer the tobacco is in place, the longer it will be before you sense a need for additional nicotine. This is in direct contrast to cigarette smoking, where the level of nicotine in the blood drops quickly when the cigarette is finished.

Miscellaneous Tips

You'll probably find that you need far fewer applications of smokeless tobacco during a typical day than you did cigarettes. While the nicotine is absorbed more slowly from these products, it will stay in your bloodstream much longer than it did in your cigarette smoking past. You will soon find yourself taking in your required nicotine fixes at longer intervals that better fit the rhythm of your day.

Do not deny yourself. All other quit-smoking programs require you to quit nicotine, and that creates a lot of dreadful feelings. I have to emphasize to switchers that this program only requires that you change the delivery system; denial and withdrawal are not included.

If you are trying to kick your nicotine addiction, by all means begin with this switch to smokeless tobacco. But get comfortable before you try cutting down or quitting altogether. If you relapse, I want you to relapse to smokeless, which reduces your health risks. Cutting down on cigarettes or switching to "low tar and nicotine" brands, as explained before, are dangerous deceptions that keep you pouring noxious fumes into your system.

121

To insure success, take the time to make your switch to smokeless tobacco as pleasurable as possible. To lessen any shock of the new, sample many products and flavors.

If you are a heavy smoker, don't be tempted to start your day with a Camel or two, telling yourself that you'll switch to snuff after breakfast. Stay consistently smokeless. If you need a kickstart of nicotine, try two pouches or some loose snuff. The particle size of these products is such that they pack easily and have less of a tendency to wander about the mouth. The least convenient of the products are those that are finely cut or ground; they are the most difficult to hold in place. However, with practice, any of these products can be managed with a minimum of trouble.

Evidence That This Method Works

You may be wondering to yourself about the chances of successfully kicking cigarettes with a switch to smokeless tobacco. You are probably thinking too much instead of going out there and getting your first can of snuff and asking questions such as "This sounds like a great theory, but can it be done? Is it possible, after all these years, after all those attempts to quit in the past, that I can stop smoking overnight and switch to smokeless tobacco? Has it been done before?" The answer to all of your questions is: "Absolutely yes!"

Despite the distorted picture of smokeless tobacco portrayed by some members of the public health establishment, there is evidence that millions of smokers have decided for themselves that smokeless tobacco is a safer alternative to cigarette smoking. Various government agencies conduct health interview surveys which collect information on what tobacco products people use. Buried deeply within these surveys is information that as many as 5.3 million people now use smokeless tobacco in the United States. The United States Government's Centers for Disease Control and Prevention estimates that 1.76 million people who use smokeless tobacco are former smokers. These people have made a decision which will impact the quality and length of their lives, and in most cases they have made it without the guidance or support of anyone in the health professions. I'm hoping that many of you will forgo the expensive hypnotists or gimmicky products and join in this effective and pleasurable way to quit smoking.

Many former smokers have told us their stories. We informally refer to these individuals as "switchers." You may find what we have learned from them of some interest and application to your particular situation. The average age of switchers is 50, but some are as young as 27 and some as old as 77. They come from all walks of life: blue and white collar, women and men. Their cigarette smoking experience varies considerably. The average smoking history involves 48 pack-years. (Pack-years is a measure of exposure to cigarettes which is obtained by multiplying the number of packs you smoke daily by the number of years that you have smoked.) Some people had recognized early on that cigarette smoking was a future health threat — they had only three pack-years. Others made the switch with an astounding 156 pack-years behind them.

Why did these people switch? Many had actually started experiencing health problems. Of these, lung and breathing problems were most common, but heart attacks were also reported as an event that definitely focused smokers' thinking on the subject. Other switchers, especially younger individuals, perceived that health problems were only a matter of time.

The switch to smokeless tobacco was no short-lived fad. The average length of time since the switch was nine years, with a range of three to fifteen years. A final bit of good news: the switchers that we talked to had no problem making the change. They were not troubled by the physical withdrawal symptoms and mental anguish normally accompanying a quit-smoking effort. They made the change easily and rapidly, and, most importantly, they made the change on their own, which all experts agree is the most effective and lasting way to quit.

Profiles of Switchers

The people depicted below are real pioneers. They are former smokers who, for various and sometimes very personal reasons, decided on their own, without any medical assistance or support, that smokeless tobacco was a safer alternative to cigarette smoking. These profiles in courage can serve as models for those of you who may be impressed by the facts, the statistics, and the logic in this book, but who need a personal touch to bring the book's message to heart.

Each one of the former smokers below has shared his or her personal story with me and my colleagues. As I share their stories with you, allow me to screen their names to protect their privacy.

Clint is a 55-year-old manager of maintenance operations for a national transportation firm. He started smoking when he was seventeen years old, and consistently smoked a pack of cigarettes a day for the next 34 years. Clint had occasionally tried to quit. In 1985, he successfully quit smoking for an extended period of time, but eventually found himself again smoking up to two packs per day.

In August 1988, Clint started experiencing pain in his lower chest and stomach area. When it did not go away, he decided to drive to the hospital for evaluation. To calm his nerves on the way, he had what turned out to be his last cigarette. Clint was suffering a heart attack.

During his hospitalization the doctors were blunt. Smoking was a big factor in the attack. To continue to smoke was to run the risk of another attack — one that might not be as mild. For Clint this was enough of an incentive to quit for good. However, the need to smoke persisted. He seemed to be longing for nicotine every minute of every hour of every day. Finally, after a year and a half of continuous craving, he started using smokeless tobacco.

Clint's story is not uncommon from several standpoints. First, a health problem resulting from smoking made a sudden appearance. Second, he continued to experience a nicotine craving long after he quit and long after the physical effects of nicotine were out of his system. This is not unusual. Many smokers enrolled in our program have quit in the past for as many as several years, but the need for nicotine did not subside. Smokeless tobacco had completely satisfied that craving.

Clint is also far luckier than the over 400,000 people who die every year from a smoking-related illness. He received a fair warning — a heart attack that wasn't fatal. Many smokers don't get the warning but suffer the massive heart attack first, the one from which they don't recover. Many smoking-induced cancers act the same way. Because they arise deep within the body, the cancers are difficult or impossible to detect early. By the time they are discovered, they are difficult or impossible to treat successfully.

Are smokers able to quit even if they see the handwriting on the wall? Many are not. As I said earlier, as many as 50 percent of smokers who have a heart attack cannot quit. The lung disease clinics are full of emphysema patients who are slowly smothering themselves cigarette by cigarette.

Carl is a retired machinist who remembers smoking when he was ten years old. For 40 years he averaged two packs a day. He smoked unfiltered Camel cigarettes for 30 years, but switched to a filtered brand when he started to experience breathing problems. When his breathing started to get considerably worse, Carl consulted a doctor. The diagnosis: emphysema. The solution: stop smoking. The outcome if he didn't: a maddeningly slow death by suffocation. Carl made the decision to quit. He tried prescription nicotine gum, but it was of no help. He knew he had to try something else soon or he would break down and resume smoking. He tried smokeless tobacco.

That was twelve years ago. His lung deterioration was slowed, and, most importantly, he is convinced that without smokeless tobacco he would still be smoking, or be six feet under.

Carl might have saved his health much earlier, but he fell into another common trap. He switched to a filtered cigarette, thinking that it would be safer, but, as established here, filters only benefit the cigarette companies. They are made of cheaper materials than tobacco, allowing the manufacturers to use less tobacco per cigarette. Are smokers really benefiting from filtered smoke? No. To get the amount of nicotine they need they are puffing harder and longer, taking in the thousands of dangerous pollutants in the smoke. Small wonder that Carl's lung symptoms did not improve with these "healthier" cigarettes.

Marian is a 77-year-old who smoked a pack of cigarettes every three or four days for decades. When she was 72 she developed a cough that scared her. As an active grandmother she never felt that her age had earned her the right to be reckless. Looking for a way to continue enjoying tobacco without harming her grandchildren (even by bad example), she hit upon the idea of trying discreet little packets of moist snuff. For the past five years Marian has been successfully substituting smokeless tobacco for cigarettes, and can't remember where she used to keep all those messy ashtrays and dangerous butane lighters.

Marian emphasizes another important point: it's never too late to quit. As I've mentioned earlier in this chapter, quitting the cigarette habit at any age leads to decreased risks for essentially all smoking-related illnesses. Smokers of Marian's age often tell me they think it's too late to quit, but they are only saying this as a defense mechanism. They cannot deny that there might be real health benefits; they know very well — often from previous painful experiences — what quitting means. Just the thought of living without nicotine is overwhelming. But only old dogs can't learn new tricks, and for smokers of all ages there is only one quit-smoking solution that does the trick — smokeless tobacco.

Wendell is a 50-year-old farm manager. He had smoked non-filtered cigarettes for fourteen years when, at the young age of 35, he started experiencing severe shortness of breath, a bad cough, and numerous sinus infections. Wendell thought he could beat these problems by switching to a pipe, but he fell into a common trap for cigarette smokers who switch to cigars or a pipe. Because a cigarette smoker gets used to the nicotine jolt obtained through inhaling the smoke, the tendency is to continue inhaling when smoking a cigar or pipe. *No smoke is healthy*, and cigar and pipe smoke can be very irritating when inhaled.

After six years of pipe smoking, Wendell decided he'd better quit altogether. After just one week of climbing the walls, he went back to the tobacco aisle and tried smokeless tobacco. Today, fifteen years later, Wendell remains smoke-free and cough-free.

Rick is 52 years old and works as a technician for a major electronics manufacturer. He started smoking when he was twenty, and for the next 29 years he consistently consumed between two and four packs a day. Rick had several close calls with another "occupational risk" of the habit. He had dozed off several times with a cigarette in his hand, coming very close to starting a major house fire. (Each year in the United States, smoking is the cause of fires that kill 1,300 people.)

Rick tried to quit tobacco altogether when he quit smoking. But he frequently craved the nicotine he was missing, even though he got over the queasy disorientation of the physical withdrawal symptoms within the first week.

After three months of constant craving, he started using smokeless tobacco. For the past three years he has been sleeping better, knowing that he won't wake up with a problem in his lungs or a burning cigarette in his hand.

Dan is a 38-year-old noncommissioned officer in the Army. He started smoking when he was sixteen years old. After smoking two packs per day for twelve years, Dan started developing shortness of breath. He made an overnight switch to smokeless tobacco.

Like many successful participants in my quit-smoking program, Dan did not experience a moment of physical or psychological withdrawal after giving up his cigarette habit. He had not read about the relative safety of smokeless tobacco, but he intuitively knew that it had to be healthier than pouring fumes into his body.

Dan has another reason today to feel great about his decision ten years ago. As you may have heard, the Department of Defense is jumping on the antismoking bandwagon with sweeping restrictions on the habit.

John is a 66-year-old who owns a small business. He had been smoking three packs of cigarettes per day for 52 years. Four years ago, doctors told him that he had hardening of the arteries, a blood vessel condition that is complicated by smoking. He switched to smokeless tobacco as soon as he realized, to his surprise, that dipping snuff gave him the same satisfaction he got from cigarettes.

John is a great example of another advantage of smokeless tobacco: it doesn't matter how much or how little you smoke, the nicotine content and the efficiency of absorption allow you to make the switch easily. You can find the right product and brand of smokeless tobacco to match any kind of cigarette you are used to.

Dr. Lee R. is a health professional in rural Alabama. He started smoking when he was twenty years old, smoking one and a half packs per day for 26 years. Like many other smokers, his entire breathing apparatus started to rebel. Dr. R. started wheezing, especially at night. In addition, he had shortness of breath, a persistent cough, and irritated sinuses and eyes. Dr. R.'s medical training had not been forgotten; these were ominous signs of more serious problems ahead if he didn't quit. He quit for three months, suffering continuous craving like so many other former smokers. Then he discovered smokeless tobacco, and for the last ten years he has been looking and feeling better.

Dr. R. has tried to convince smoking friends and relatives to make the switch. He worked on his brother for years, but was not able to convince him to make the transition. His brother has since died from lung cancer.

James P. is a magazine editor who had been smoking one pack of cigarettes daily for 38 of his 54 years. When he went for his yearly physical ten years ago, a test showed that his lungs were rapidly losing capacity. He decided that it was time to quit. He tried both the nicotine gum and patch, but was not satisfied with either. James went back and complained to his pharmacist. Imagine a conversation like this:

"Well, Mr. P., we have some smokeless tobacco products up front that you could try."

"Smokeless tobacco? To put inside my mouth? Do I look like a cowboy to you?"

"My wife settled on four or five pouches of snuff a day, and she's no cowboy."

James ended up a healthier man, having switched to a brand of snuff that did not evoke the Old West at all. Nevertheless, the pharmacist has not stopped calling him "Cowboy."

Now ask yourself if you are so very different from these people. If these veteran smokers could try something different, but something that delivered the same tobacco pleasure they needed, so could you. It's a win-win situation. Your loved ones will think you are a brave hero for giving up cigarettes, but you'll be smiling on the inside, drawing in all the tobacco flavor you desire.

Meet Some Switchers

Try to find out who has switched in your neighborhood, on your job, or at your church. Chances are good that people will be happy to share their success stories with you. You might even inquire with a friendly salesperson where you buy your tobacco. Someone reaching for a can of Bandits while you are hovering around the tobacco shelf may also be a good source of information.

Switchers everywhere have accepted that they need tobacco. You won't get a nasty lecture about quitting from someone who has merely made a logical compromise. Try a line like, "How are those packets of snuff compared to cigarettes? Are you a former smoker?" Most switchers are true believers, and you will probably get friendly advice and inspiration.

Secondhand Smokeless

In Chapter Four I discussed secondhand smoke. I emphasized that there is no such thing as secondhand saliva, but there is a very real and important phenomenon that I will call secondhand smokeless. The resulting condition is actually quite contagious. You see, it starts with a few brave pioneers finding a gap through the Smoky Mountains of damning medical evidence. Once they have left Marlboro Country and crossed the frontier into healthy and pleasurable smokeless tobacco, they attract whole wagon-trains full of friends and relatives to follow their trail.

It is hoped that this book opens up a whole populous state of switchers, where now there is only a smokeless tobacco territory. The only viable hope for the last 46 million smokers in this country is this painless "smokeless solution" that has not received any publicity (Unless you are counting the undeserved negative rap that smokeless tobacco has received in the media's anti-Salem witch trials against the cigarette manufacturers.) Once the United States, and eventually the world, gets the facts straight, even big city folks on the east and west coasts will not mistake smokeless tobacco for something a Southerner chews or a baseball player spits when cigarettes aren't convenient.

With sanitary and discreet pouches of flavorful snuff, the smokeless tobacco industry has come a long way since the days of the chaw and spittoon. This new set of products will allow smokers to live longer through adaptation. Let a neat pouch of snuff replace those burning coffin nails, and let tobacco slowly fade away without a trail of smoke.

~ ~ ~

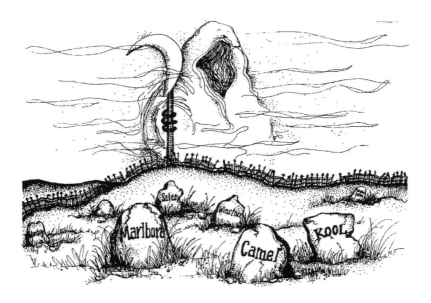

Chapter Eight
Politics and Pragmatism

Chapter Eight
Politics and Pragmatism

*Fanaticism consists of redoubling your effort
when you have forgotten your aim.*

— George Santayana (1863-1952)

Why Hasn't This Book Been Written Before?

The thesis of this book is so new that it will undoubtedly be controversial. The medical information on which the book is based, on the other hand, is not entirely new. I have (quite modestly I might add) quoted key research that we have conducted here at the University of Alabama at Birmingham, but the original data charting the (remarkably low) rate of oral cancer among smokeless tobacco users was published in the New England Journal of Medicine in 1981. Since then, several other published studies in the mid-1980's have supported the accuracy of the original data.

This important research has been studied and its facts have been accepted as valid by thousands of researchers, but they permitted their biases to cloud their interpretation, and they failed to see the contrast between the health effects of cigarette smoking and those of smokeless tobacco use. Therefore, the most useful perspective was never publicized, and, sadly, smokers have lost many precious years worth of opportunities to switch to healthier smokeless tobacco products. I write this book with all the more urgency to allow those uninformed smokers the chance to keep enjoying tobacco without suffering from deadly and debilitating diseases.

What is the answer to the question posed in the subtitle above? This book was not written earlier because of the stalemate in the tobacco war. Virtually every group on both sides of the smoking issue contributes to the current deadlock in the tobacco debate — and opposes the introduction of the humane and logical smokeless tobacco solution. You would think that the tobacco industry would grab at the smokeless tobacco concept as a way to save the industry from drowning. But no, they seem happy to be treading water and claiming that the water isn't over their heads at all. The antitobacco fanatics have gone off the deep end, too. My program, if completely implemented, would result in a 98 percent reduction in tobacco-related deaths. Yet it has already been labelled as bad public health policy.

It is important for us to examine this status quo in the tobacco war. Billions of dollars and even bigger egos are on the line. The cigarette barons, with the best lawyers and politicians that money can buy, war with the antismoking activists, armed with opinions of health professionals and badges of political correctness. As the battle lines on smoking have been drawn in our society over the past 30 years, it is clear that one thing has been forgotten by both the pro- and antitobacco warriors: the American smoker.

The Cigarette Manufacturers

First, let's look at the cigarette manufacturers. Earlier this century, cigarette makers were like any other industry competing for the loose change of the American public, ever searching for the best product to mass produce, distribute, and sell. The Marlboro man wandered into tombstone territory when the trickle of health warnings about smoking in the 1940's and 1950's turned into a flood of knowledge in the past two decades. Today, the basic facts are undeniable: cigarette smoking is a risky activity. Even in the face of these facts, the cigarette manufacturers persist in defending their products. They continually deny that their products, when used as intended, produce the dreaded diseases that I have relentlessly cataloged throughout this book.

On one level, this mule-like stubbornness on the part of Joe Camel is readily transparent. Like many other companies, cigarette makers' sole purpose is to make money for themselves and their shareholders, and ethics be damned. The territorial advances of the antismokers — the constraints placed upon cigarette advertising, the taxes on cigarette sales, and the limitation of public smoking — have been successfully absorbed by the armies of the Carolinas and Virginias. For effect, though, each of these small victories was won over the cries and howls of the cigarette manufacturers.

The tobacco forces don't mind little defeats at all. Survival in this war means victory and vast profits in each quarter. There are very good reasons for their seemingly ridiculous denial of adverse health effects. For a moment, let's imagine that the manufacturers admitted that cigarette smoking is in some way causally related to lung cancer. Would this be calling a truce or total surrender? In our litigious society it would be suicide. The tobacco industry would immediately be engulfed in liability lawsuits. As the first case is decided in favor of the plaintiffs, all industry assets and future earnings would be ripe pickings for huge financial awards.

Like the asbestos industry a decade ago, the cigarette manufacturers would have to bail out, and all cigarette production would cease. We would be left with only one small problem: 46 million tobacco addicts with no possible way to service their addiction. Although the forced elimination of tobacco products has immediate intuitive appeal, beware of any solution with the scent of prohibition.

Cigarette manufacturers have used two basic strategies in battling the antitobacco zealots. The first is to argue that tobacco represents an economically important industry of vital national concern. The tobacco lobby is fond of saying that elimination of tobacco use in this country would jeopardize the livelihood of 600,000 farmers who produce this country's annual crop, as well as the jobs of countless others involved in the processing, manufacturing, distribution, and marketing steps. To hear these arguments one would assume that the tobacco industry is right up there with the auto industry. As goes Philip Morris, so goes the nation.

In reality, these jobs are concentrated in only 51 of the nation's 531 congressional districts and are a major factor in only 27. However, these are conservative districts that elect lifetime representatives with the political longevity to climb to high positions of authority within Congress. You don't find young, reforming politicians in the tobacco states — for very long. The deep drawling veterans of Marlboro country don't let Washington forget the many votes and dollars they represent.

The second defense strategy of the cigarette manufacturers is to argue that cigarette smoking is essentially a freedom of choice issue. While there is some foundation to this argument, one can counter that nicotine, and any true addiction, limits the freedom of the user.

Whose Freedom of Choice?

The proposal put forth in this book addresses this last point explicitly. I would agree completely that the use of tobacco by adults is a freedom of choice issue. (Not so, however, with the use of tobacco by children. All facets of our society are morally obligated to prevent tobacco addiction from being established in children.)

I am concerned here with the 46 million American adults who are addicted to tobacco, regardless of how they became imprisoned. Once an individual is addicted, where is his or her freedom of choice? Within the narrow cell of nicotine addiction there is a painless way to break out to a better, minimum security facility. This book is a cake with a saw inside to help you make that escape. You can eat your cake (enjoying tobacco) without the ostracizing and guilt of smoking. The minimum-risk alternative of smokeless tobacco is like a work-release program — no one will know that you are still imprisoned.

The Antitobacco Movement

What about the antitobacco troopers? Being on the "health" side of this conflict, have they acted with any more honor than their corporate counterparts? The answer appears to be "no," and precisely because they have increasingly treated the issue as a moral crusade. Russell Baker, in his "Observer" column in the *New York Times*, recently commented upon the antismoking fervor. He suggested that "crusades typically start by being admirable, proceed to being foolish, and end by being dangerous." He characterized the current tobacco holy war as entering the dangerous stage.

The tobacco reformers have dusted off the dangerous triad of weapons called regulation, legislation, and litigation in their attempt to indiscriminately eradicate tobacco use.

The *New England Journal of Medicine* published an article in April 1994 outlining the "essential components of a campaign to prevent tobacco use." Note the prohibitionist language in that phrase, and check out the stockpile of weapons to be used in this attack:

1. Increased federal excise taxes.

2. Comprehensive restrictions on smoking in the workplace and in public.

3. Bans on advertising and sponsorship by tobacco companies.

4. Comprehensive and enforced restrictions on sales of tobacco to minors.

5. Limitation of tobacco-crop subsidies.

6. Government support for conversion of tobacco crops to other crops.

7. Financial support for tobacco counter-advertising.

8. Enhanced community education programs.

9. Divestment of tobacco company stocks by universities and public institutions.

10. Support for personal injury litigation against the tobacco industry.

11. Physician-supervised counseling on smoking cessation.

First, let me point out that I wholeheartedly support restrictions on public smoking, provided that they are based on sound scientific principles and are levied fairly. I unequivocally support the restriction of tobacco sales to minors, as I have stated several times elsewhere in this book. Eighty to ninety percent of smokers start when they are teenagers. Currently 46 states have outlawed the sale of tobacco products to minors, but compliance is abysmal. Tobacco initiation is a serious issue.

However, in addition to these two items, the only other strategies discussed in that article are bans on advertising and tobacco subsidies and tobacco taxes. In other words, while education programs are only mentioned for effect, the big guns in the antismoking arsenal are those involving big government. In the rush to regulation, the fanatics have forgotten the value of education, which is the foundation of the smokeless tobacco solution.

The smokeless tobacco solution puts you, the smoker, back in control of the tobacco debate. It doesn't involve restrictions, taxation, bans, litigation, or prohibition. Besides, the prohibitionists are dreaming. Tobacco has enjoyed wide popularity in every culture into which it has been introduced over the past 500 years. Tobacco prohibition isn't simply oppressive; it won't work, and the crusaders know it.

In pursuit of a tobacco-free nirvana, the fanatics don't exactly have a perfect record. The percentage of smokers in the United States has dropped, but at 46 million, the country is far from smoke-free. Modern antismoking efforts, at first glance, may appear to have been major victories for antismoking activists, but the outcome is more complex when examined by sober, retrospective analysis.

Chapter Two's story ended with the Surgeon General's Report on Cigarette Smoking in 1964. The report, largely an educational effort, single-handedly cut cigarette sales that year by 2 percent. It also triggered full frontal assaults, including advertising restrictions, warning label requirements, and passive smoking legislation.

The Government Made Us Do It, But We Told You So

In 1966, the first health warnings were placed on cigarettes. The Federal Trade Commission had wanted tougher language, but the cigarette barons called in some favors from legislators to get the language softened, i.e., no words (perhaps the most effective) like "cancer" and "death." Still, this was a start. From the standpoint of public education, it might have been a great victory, but the warnings had one unexpected result.

After January 1, 1966, smokers could no longer claim ignorance when their personal smoking time bomb went off and they looked for somebody to blame. The warning labels provided the industry with a safe shelter, which is largely intact to this day, against product liability lawsuits.

The Government Made Us Do It, and We Screamed All the Way To the Bank

In 1968 an attorney named John Banzhaf declared guerilla warfare on cigarette advertising. During the 1950's and 1960's, cigarette companies had been spending tremendous amounts of money on television ads, and Banzhaf petitioned the government for the right to run free antismoking ads. His strategy was based on the Fairness Doctrine, a somewhat obscure law which dictated that on matters of great public importance, both sides of an issue must be fairly represented in the broadcast media. His position was that, since cigarette ads presented only one side of an important issue, antismoking commercials should be broadcast to provide balance. Moreover, the broadcasters would have to provide the air time free of charge.

From 1968 to 1970, despite howls of protest from the tobacco industry (and initially the networks), one free antismoking ad was broadcast for every three cigarette commercials. Cigarette consumption actually dropped. Then the cigarette barons got smart and the howling stopped. The tobacco companies agreed to a total broadcast ban.

Wait a minute. A total ban, effective on January 1, 1971, had to be a big victory for antismoking groups. At the time there was much rejoicing, but the ban had other far-reaching and unanticipated effects.

First, the ban saved the cigarette makers quite a bit of money on television advertising, which for many years had been viewed as an ineffective but necessary money drain. The companies didn't take this windfall to the bank; they simply redirected the money to print media like newspapers and magazines, which were — not coincidentally — considered far more cost-effective. Money talks, and many magazines don't run stories that alienate advertisers and dry up ad revenues. In this way the cigarette barons leveraged the broadcast ban into major editorial clout in the print media.

The excess cash also fueled diversification. The tobacco companies increased purchases of and mergers with a host of firms, with many previously prominent tobacco names disappearing behind layers of corporate entities with more legitimate consumer products and services. The antitobacco forces could no longer aim their missiles at easily identified tobacco company targets. These moves also enhanced the editorial domination of print media. If a magazine was scheduled to run an antismoking article, tobacco barons could pull an entire package of food and beverage ads in addition to tobacco, creating a big gash in advertising revenues.

The antismoking ads were off the tube, too. Or at least almost. With the Fairness Doctrine no longer in effect, the crusaders had to start paying for the ads. The number of ads plummeted, their effect was lost, and cigarette sales were soon on the rebound.

The FDA Plan: Make Nicotine Addiction Fade Away

A group of tobacco reformers, led by Food and Drug Administration Commissioner Dr. David Kessler, has a new regulatory strategy: reduce the amount of nicotine in cigarettes gradually over a ten to fifteen year period. The theory is that at the end of this period the nicotine concentration of cigarettes will be too low to allow nicotine addiction to be established in new smokers. In the meantime the strategy is intended to serve as a (mandatory) national withdrawal program for the nation's current 46 million smokers.

The opening volley in this regulatory power play was fired by Kessler in February 1994 in a letter to the Coalition on Smoking or Health. He announced his intention to consider regulating cigarettes as a drug delivery system for nicotine. The FDA has broad regulatory authority over foods and food additives, drugs, chemicals, and cosmetics, as stipulated by the Food, Drug and Cosmetic Act of 1938. This legislation defines a drug as "an article (other than food) intended to affect the structure or function of the body." As I discussed in Chapter Five, nicotine has well documented effects on virtually every organ system in the body, so there is no problem with this part of Kessler's rationale.

In order to regulate tobacco, the FDA also needs to show "that cigarette makers have the ability to control levels of nicotine — that speaks to the issue of intent," according to Kessler. Throughout the first half of 1994, Kessler maintained that the FDA was only on a fact-finding mission, but he also added that the evidence suggests that the cigarette manufacturers are "behaving like pharmaceutical companies."

Kessler has collaborators in this regulatory quest at the highest levels of academia and government. Two well known experts on nicotine addiction, Dr. Neal Benowitz from the University of California at San Francisco and Dr. Jack Henningfield from the National Institute on Drug Abuse, wrote an editorial in the *New England Journal of Medicine* essentially endorsing Kessler's plan. Although they admitted that "a threshold for nicotine addiction is a theoretical concept ....," these researchers still postulated a safe concentration of nicotine in cigarettes that would prevent addiction in new smokers. To reach this level, the FDA would have to order a reduction in nicotine content from about eight milligrams per cigarette to about one-half of a milligram, representing a 94 percent reduction.

Although Kessler's idea has not been tested with regard to prevention, his plan has been studied for many years as a smoking cessation option. It is basically a drawn-out variation of a strategy called nicotine fading, in which the smoker's exposure to nicotine is gradually reduced to very low levels. The concept was first introduced in 1979, and numerous trials, usually combining nicotine fading with other behavioral modifications, were conducted throughout the 1980's.

In a recent review of 21 different quit-smoking strategies, nicotine fading came in with a success rate that will not surprise readers of this book — about 25 percent. Dr. Michael C. Fiore, director of the Center for Tobacco Research and Intervention at the University of Wisconsin, questioned the effectiveness of this strategy in helping current smokers quit. Of course if Dr. Kessler has his way, this program will not be optional. In other words, a large percentage of current smokers may not find this forced nicotine withdrawal a pleasant experience. What will they do?

As they did with low tar low nicotine cigarettes and those with filters, smokers will initially respond to Kessler's nicotine phase-out plan by smoking more often and more intensely. Benowitz and Henningfield acknowledged this problem in their editorial. They responded by saying that these smokers' "short-term (ten-year) risk may be offset by the long-term benefit of a greater likelihood that they will quit smoking (as cigarettes become less satisfying) and by the enormous benefit of preventing nicotine addiction in future generations." In other words, they are sorry if your risks increase for ten years because you can't quit, but maybe you'll quit anyway and besides, maybe your children won't get hooked.

Another drawback to Kessler's plan is its potential to spawn another huge illicit drug problem. He has commented that "even if we don't ban cigarettes, we could create a black market by removing the nicotine too quickly." He seems to believe that the problem is avoidable simply by reducing the nicotine slowly. He is undaunted: "We need to withdraw it at just the right pace, letting the addiction fade as we reduce the nicotine."

There are other fundamental problems with Kessler's strategy. For example, setting a threshold level of nicotine exposure below which it is not addictive is an extremely speculative tactic. This would imply that there may be a "safe" level of consumption for all addictions including alcohol, cocaine, and heroin. Our caffeine comparison from Chapter Five also serves us well here. Utilizing the same rationale concerning effect on body function (addictive potential) and intent (ability to manipulate levels), the FDA has ruled that caffeine is a food additive at concentrations up to 0.02 percent. This amounts to 72 milligrams of caffeine in a twelve-ounce soda. The FDA designates over-the-counter products containing caffeine (up to 200 milligrams per dose) as stimulants. Consistency is not a strong feature of the FDA's caffeine policy, because a twelve-ounce serving of coffee can have as much as 400 milligrams of caffeine.

The important lesson from the caffeine analysis is that the FDA can draw on a precedent for every aspect of the nicotine fading strategy. Kessler's plan seems to be bolstered by an elegant scientific rationale, and it superficially appears to be a new and creative approach to the problem of nicotine addiction. However, that's where the real problem lies. Because antitobacco groups have passed judgement on nicotine addiction, they have focused all of their energy on eradicating tobacco. The nicotine fade is simply a thinly veiled disguise for tobacco prohibition.

The Tax Conundrum

Another familiar battle cry recently has been "Bring on the sin taxes." The reasons: excise taxes will reduce consumption and the revenue generated can be used to pay for increased costs of governmental health programs and medical research. These rationales merit closer examination, because the government must choose one to the exclusion of the other.

If the government's goal is to decrease consumption, then kiss revenue generation good-bye. Reducing cigarette smoking is certainly a laudable goal, but why not apply excise taxes with surgical precision, which provides economic incentives for smokers contemplating the switch to smokeless tobacco.

When it comes to excise taxes, I have a strong suspicion that the national government has one goal: revenue generation. In other words, the federal government has dollar signs, not vital signs, on its agenda. The first American excise tax on tobacco was part of the Internal Revenue Act of 1864. Was this a benevolent attempt to save the health of the American tobacco user? Hardly. The government needed a way out of the deficit created by the Civil War.

Keep in mind that, because the ultimate goal of taxation is the transfer or redistribution of wealth, the government singles out for excise taxes only those products for which there are no ready substitutes. Witness gasoline, tobacco, and alcohol. Polls currently indicate that Americans favor increasing excise taxes on cigarettes by a margin of three to one, which should surprise no one. That's the ratio of nonsmokers to smokers. If you're a nonsmoker and are waxing enthusiastic over the prospect of increased cigarette taxes, take stock of the products and activities that you enjoy. The precedents set today by tobacco taxes can be applied to your favorite products in the not too distant future.

How Smokeless Tobacco Gets Chewed Up and Spat Out By the Media

In the war over tobacco, the smokeless solution has been trapped in no-man's land. When smoking came under attack as a cause of disease in the 1960's and 1970's, smokeless tobacco companies recognized an opportunity to promote their products as a safer alternative to cigarettes. They launched massive advertising campaigns in the late 1970's and early 1980's which were effective, resulting in increased smokeless tobacco sales.

In response, the antitobacco crusaders redirected their media missiles at smokeless tobacco, using the unreasonable and impractical "no safe alternative" tactic detailed in Chapter Seven. In 1986 Congress passed the Smokeless Tobacco Health Education Act, which formalized the federal government's position against smokeless tobacco and banned its broadcast advertising. The antismokeless campaign has greatly influenced not only the public's perception of smokeless tobacco, but the views of medical experts nationwide. For example, in 1990, Prevention magazine surveyed 200 leading experts from the 44 National Cancer Institute designated cancer centers concerning ways for individuals to reduce their cancer risks. Ninety-nine percent of the experts agreed that the best cancer prevention measure was to avoid smoking or chewing tobacco.

In the Media Spotlight

After several years of research, I published my concept for the smokeless tobacco solution in professional medical and scientific journals in July 1994. As a result, I was invited to present my plan on *Good Morning America*. Dr. Greg Connolly, Director of the Massachusetts Tobacco Control Program, was invited to respond to my plan on the same program. Dr. Connolly's comments provide excellent insight into the nonscientific responses to my smokeless tobacco solution. Judge for yourself the extent to which Dr. Connolly employs a scientific basis for opposing the smokeless tobacco solution.

First, Dr. Connolly started out with a charming definition: "Tobacco is tobacco is tobacco whether you chew it, smoke it, or put it in your mouth." He then launched into an emotional but inaccurate comparison of smoking and smokeless tobacco use: "You significantly increase your risk for mouth cancer. So what you are doing basically is you're trading body parts, one cancer for the other." However, Dr. Connolly did not point out that for smokers who switch, "increased risk" isn't in the vocabulary, and any trade of risks is definitely *down* for *every* tobacco-related disease.

My solution does not require tobacco abstinence. To zealots this is committing the ultimate tobacco sin, so Dr. Connolly moved to ethical issues: "I would just point out from a medical ethics perspective I don't know anybody, any physician or dentist in this country that would turn to a smoker who couldn't quit and say 'I am going to write you a prescription for a known cancer causing agent while we have nicotine replacement therapy such as patches that we can prescribe.'" Since my plan offers the smoker a 98 percent reduction in the risk of a tobacco-related death, it obviously meets the highest ethical standards. Dr. Connolly will soon be meeting lots of physicians and dentists recommending the switch to smokeless. By the way, no prescription is necessary.

Then he questioned the medical publishing process: "But let me point out that the article was an editorial, it was an opinion of one individual. It was not the opinion of the journal." Every article in every medical journal is the work of the authors. The scientific accuracy of my article, which Dr. Connolly did not question, was rigorously double checked by the journal editors and reviewers in a process called peer review. Along with Dr. Philip Cole, an epidemiologist, I subsequently published additional supporting research in *Nature*, a prestigious scientific journal.

Dr. Connolly made the obvious observation that others haven't endorsed my program: "When every major health organization in this country has looked at the issue and carefully weighed the evidence, the American Dental Association, the National Cancer Institute, the World Health Organization. Every organization has said smokeless tobacco is not a safe alternative to cigarette smoking." Looking at the issue is not necessarily the same as carefully weighing the evidence, as Dr. Connolly himself has demonstrated. As an alternative to cigarette smoking, smokeless tobacco is not perfectly safe, it is just *98 percent* less dangerous.

Next, he trivialized tobacco use by comparing it to jumping from tall buildings: He said that switching from smoking to the use of smokeless tobacco is "like jumping from a third floor versus the tenth floor. And it is something that health professionals don't advocate." If I must continue the analogy, I would point out that switchers are not jumping from any window, they are taking the stairs.

Finally, Dr. Connolly returned to an ethical attack: "To tell someone they can develop a mouth cancer in lieu of a lung cancer really raises many serious ethical concerns and for a physician or a dentist to prescribe that to a patient ...I would say I would check my malpractice...If that person does develop mouth cancer and turns back to the dentist and says 'gee doc you told me to quit smoking now I've got mouth cancer what do I do?' I would have a pretty good lawyer." I agree that there is an ethical concern. But it is the reverse of Dr. Connolly's view. Since smokeless tobacco users live eight years longer than smokers, it is absolutely unethical to continue to deny smokers information that could save their lives.

Notice that Dr. Connolly tried to deal with ethics and the legitimacy of the idea, but in his tirade, Dr. Connolly never disputed the solid scientific data and logic on which this book is based. Dr. Connolly's views are very representative of the strong emotional reaction that the smokeless tobacco solution elicits from antitobacco crusaders. There may be a number of reasons for this: the crusaders are not aware of the scientific facts that I have scrupulously assembled to support my solution; they are aware of the facts but are unable to interpret them correctly, or more likely; the antitobacco crusade has entered a stage where scientific facts are simply ignored as irrelevant.

The antitobacco movement is understandably frustrated by the current impasse in reducing the annual death toll related to smoking. This frustration also comes from the fact that the movement has not been able to respond to the impasse with new ideas. And so they have turned in desperation to regulatory and legislative methods of tobacco control. These ultimately emerge as variations on one theme: prohibition.

If you think that Connolly's comments are unusually denigrating, be advised that they are coming from an activist whose views on tobacco are clear, though unimaginative and inflexible. He has published his solution for smokeless tobacco, at least for Europe.

In a 1991 letter to *The Lancet*, a respected British medical journal, Connolly presented a very simple plan for the twelve European Commission countries with regard to smokeless tobacco: *Ban all products*. (Of course, this was the opinion of one person, not the opinion of the journal.)

Activists like Connolly have transformed themselves from health care professionals to advocates for tobacco elimination. To a prohibitionist, no other plan measures up. Furthermore, they are threatened by the smokeless tobacco solution because it takes the tobacco issue out of their hands, placing it squarely where it belongs, in the hands of the smoker — you.

Looking Beyond Conventional Wisdom

The deliberate confusion of the risks of smoking and smokeless tobacco has led to a highly exaggerated assessment of smokeless tobacco's health risks which has entered the sacred realm of conventional wisdom. Because journalists and general interest writers rely upon information provided by experts, it is not surprising that the nation's news media espouses the conventional wisdom that smokeless tobacco is not a safer substitute for cigarette smoking.

In October 1993, two articles appeared in the health section of the *Washington Post* under the title "Chewing Tobacco: A Baseball Tradition that Can Be Deadly." Both authors were obviously striving to be accurate in their references to smokeless tobacco. They interviewed prominent health experts, but a number of quotes from these articles demonstrate how inaccurate conventional wisdom is passed off as proven fact.

Misconception:

"Former United States Surgeon General Antonia C. Novello warned last year that the trend [of increasing smokeless tobacco use] could cause 'a full blown oral cancer epidemic two or three decades from now.'"

144

Because I do not endorse smokeless tobacco use by anyone except the smoker who wants to quit, I am also concerned with any increased use in nonsmokers, especially children. However, the statement by Dr. Novello is overly dramatic and has been blown way out of proportion. Let me place it in perspective, by proposing the absolute worst case scenario: every adult in the United States (190 million) immediately starts using smokeless tobacco. In several decades (the more accurate number is five instead of two or three), the epidemic predicted by Dr. Novello would consist of 25,000 deaths every year from smokeless tobacco-related oral cancer.

Every one of those deaths would be tragic and avoidable. But these 25,000 deaths (in 190 million smokeless tobacco users) would represent only one-sixteenth (yes, only 6.3 percent!) of the 419,000 smokers who now die every year (out of 46 million smokers).

Misconception:

"Oral cancer... is more than 50 times more common among longtime snuff users than among nonusers, according to the National Cancer Institute. About 30,000 cases are diagnosed each year..."

The relative risk of oral cancer related to smokeless tobacco use is four, not 50. To use the higher number is to deliberately distort snuff's true risks. During that *Good Morning America* appearance Dr. Connolly tried to slip the 50 figure by me and the American people. He knows better. And after reading this book, you do too.

Notice how the 30,000 annual cases of oral cancer are apparently attributed to smokeless tobacco in the second part of the quote. This is a distortion accomplished by clever writing, because the statement is absolutely correct, but what has been omitted is that about 90 percent of these 30,000 cases (or 27,400) are actually associated with smoking. If 12 million Americans are long term users (as stated earlier in the article), you could expect only 3,120 cases of oral cancer related to smokeless tobacco, which accounts for the remaining cases.

Misconception:

"[A National Cancer Institute report on smokeless tobacco] details the history of dipping and chewing and explains why they are potentially as dangerous as smoking cigarettes.

"'The biggest fallacy is that it [smokeless tobacco use] is a safe alternative to smoking,' said Jerome C. Goldstein, a physician and the executive director of the American Academy of Otolaryngology-Head and Neck Surgery. 'It certainly is not.'"

As I noted in Chapter Seven, 12,000 yearly cases of oral cancer among 46 million smokeless tobacco users would represent only one-twentieth of all smoking related cancers (230,000), less than one-tenth of smoking related lung cancers (145,300), and less than half of the number of oral cancers (27,400) now attributed to smoking. Research also suggests that smokeless tobacco use carries little or no risk for heart disease, which kills almost 180,000 smokers every year, and the threat of problems like emphysema is nonexistent.

To summarize with a direct comparison, of the 46 million American smokers, 419,000 die each year from smoking-related cancers, heart problems, and lung disease. With 46 million smokeless tobacco users, only 6,000 deaths from oral cancer would result per year.

Misconception:

"Smokers who kick their smoking habit and then trade in their cigarettes for snuff, experts say, may be merely substituting one addictive habit for another — and trading high lung-cancer risk for high oral cancer risk."

The most recent CDC survey of smokeless tobacco use indicated that one-third (between 1.5 and 2 million) of current smokeless tobacco users list themselves as former smokers. In making this switch, they have reduced their risk of heart attacks, all cancers and lung disease. They have not merely traded one habit for another. These individuals have recognized what experts and organizations have overlooked or ignored in their collective zeal to condemn all tobacco use. Smokeless tobacco use has risks, but is unquestionably much safer, resulting in far fewer and significantly less serious health risks, which are more easily managed, than cigarette smoking.

Robert Parry, an investigative reporter for the PBS series *Frontline*, has written a book entitled *Fooling America: How Washington Insiders Twist the Truth and Manufacture the Conventional Wisdom* (William Morrow and Company, New York, 1992). He argues that conventional wisdom, when based on superficial analysis and trivialization of important issues, is a barrier to the thorough debate necessary to solve the nation's most pressing problems. Although written primarily from a political and foreign policy perspective, its messages can also be applied to the nation's current debate over tobacco use.

Media discussions of tobacco use have been dominated by widely polarized, and in some ways, equally distorted positions. The cigarette manufacturers claim that health effects have never been proven. The medical experts assert that all tobacco use is equally risky. Superficial analysis and trivialization have obscured critical central facts; first, that over 1,100 Americans die each day from diseases resulting from a legal addiction with a ghastly delivery system, and second, that there is a socially compatible way to contend with the addiction that results in far fewer and less serious health problems.

Parry encourages the public and the pundits to "give a fair hearing to the fresh idea or unusual argument." This book proposes just such an idea, and its unusual argument is intended to push the debate on tobacco use past the conventional wisdom. It challenges smokers and nonsmokers alike to think about tobacco in a fundamentally different way.

A Global Epilogue

My primary concern in this book is you, the American smoker. But smoking is a worldwide phenomenon; at least 1 billion people smoke 5.2 trillion cigarettes every year. There is no reason why smokeless tobacco can't be a worldwide solution.

Smoking in many developed nations, as measured by per capita consumption, peaked sometime between the 1960's and the 1980's.

For example, consumption peaked in the United States in 1964 (after the release of the first Surgeon General's report) and in Canada in 1981. The United Kingdom topped out in 1972, and most countries in Western Europe had maximal smoking rates in the 1970's and early 1980's, followed by declining rates thereafter. Although this is good news, we must be careful about signalling the end of smoking. Firstly, although the percentage of smokers has gradually decreased in these countries, remember that the activity selects against itself by killing off its faithful practitioners. Thus, even with impressive quitting statistics and sadly more impressive death tolls, new smokers continue to fill in the ranks.

Secondly, the population has increased substantially in all these countries. Thus, even though the percentages are down, the absolute number of smokers may not have dropped; these numbers may even have risen. Cigarettes will continue to take their toll on developed countries. It has been estimated that over 20 percent of the current population in these countries will eventually die of a smoking-related illness. That translates into 250 million of the total population of 1.25 billion people in these countries.

Additional challenges remain in many international markets where demand for cigarettes is booming. Previously uncultivated markets include Asia, Africa, Latin America, Eastern Europe, and the nations which comprise the former Soviet Union. There are more smokers in China (300 million) than there are people in the entire United States.

Often this phenomenon is blamed exclusively on the aggressive marketing, cutthroat business, and unscrupulous political activities of the six transnational tobacco companies. Certainly these giants have not ignored the prospects of these enormous markets, but there are other fundamental reasons for the smoking explosion in these regions. For one, until very recently, the American government helped the tobacco companies force open foreign markets. Tobacco was once a prominent component of our government's Food For Aid program, which in essence forced our poor trading partners in need of food to take our tobacco exports as well.

These markets are also opening up on their own. For decades markets in Eastern Europe and Asia were dominated by state monopolies, which controlled the sale of about half of all the world's cigarettes. Recent political changes in these areas have resulted in the relaxation of former restrictions and the laying down of a welcome mat for the tobacco companies. And the welcome mat is woven out of only one material — money. Because, make no mistake about it, tobacco means money. Exactly 400 years after Columbus started the great transnational movement of tobacco from the North American continent, over 15 billion pounds of tobacco were grown in 117 countries.

Let me illustrate how much tobacco means to many economies, especially those of third world countries, primarily because tobacco cultivation provides them with cash, price stability, and rural employment. Looking at the Gross Domestic Product (GDP), tobacco contributes more than food and beverages combined in Bangladesh, Cuba, and Indonesia. Its share of the GDP is greater than either food or beverages in China, Ghana, Jordan, Libya, Nepal, Pakistan, and Sri Lanka. In Zaire tobacco contributes as much as food, and it outranks beverages in the Central African Republic, Mali, Somalia, and Western Samoa. For comparison, tobacco's share of the GDP in the United States is only 14 percent of food and beverages combined.

Ever wonder why governments don't do something really significant about smoking? Consider for a moment that tobacco generated at least $140 billion in taxes for governments in 1992. They recognize — although they don't readily admit it — that restrictive measures to destroy the legitimate tobacco industry would drive all this economic activity underground, demolishing the cash flow without damaging the habit. The restriction experiment has already been tried — in the United States during Prohibition — and you know the results.

Let's face it. All of these powerful forces would not be relevant if not for one unavoidable fact: using tobacco is enjoyable. The smokeless tobacco solution that is currently working for Sweden, can work for many smokers in the United States and can be exported to many countries around the globe.

In fact, there is evidence that the solution is being quietly implemented. I have examined American tobacco exports as reported by the U. S. Department of Commerce National Trade Data Bank, Economic and Statistics Administration. Its report lists the major export countries for American smokeless tobacco. I want you to grasp the trend in the table.

Major Export Countries for American Smokeless Tobacco			
1989	1990	1991	1992
Canada	Canada	Canada	Canada
Sweden	Sweden	Sweden	Sweden
Norway	Norway	Norway	Norway
Cayman Islands	Cayman Islands	Cayman Islands	Cayman Islands
Bermuda	Bermuda	Bermuda	Bermuda
	West Germany	West Germany	West Germany
	Mexico	Mexico	Mexico
			Japan
			Bahrain
			United Arab Emirates
			Saudi Arabia
			Netherlands
			Austria
			Finland
			Iceland
			Australia
			South Korea

Back in 1970, a researcher by the name of E.R. Tufte designed the interocular trauma test — the point when a researcher becomes aware of the meaning of his data because the conclusion hits him between the eyes. Hopefully, the readers of this book — smokers and nonsmokers, legislators, policy analysts, and health professionals — will take this test, and embrace the smokeless tobacco solution and its potential for worldwide distribution.

~ ~ ~

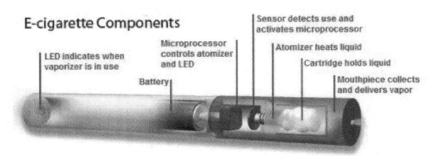

E-cigarette Components

LED indicates when vaporizer is in use

Microprocessor controls atomizer and LED

Battery

Sensor detects use and activates microprocessor

Atomizer heats liquid

Cartridge holds liquid

Mouthpiece collects and delivers vapor

(Image courtesy of National Vapers Club)

Chapter Nine
The E-Cigarette Solution

Chapter Nine
The E-Cigarette Solution

"There is little doubt that if it were not for the nicotine...people would be little more inclined to smoke than they are to blow bubbles or light sparklers."

Michael A. H. Russell. Realistic goals for
smoking and health: a case for safer smoking.
The Lancet 1, 254-258, 1974.

The e-Revolution Has Arrived

In 1995, *For Smokers Only* envisioned a new paradigm for tobacco use with minimal adverse health consequences; it was based on a large-scale conversion from combustible to smoke-free tobacco/nicotine consumption. Over the subsequent 18 years, cigarette sales declined and smokeless tobacco use steadily increased. Still, social barriers, coupled with fierce opposition from influential tobacco prohibitionists, deterred widespread adoption of safer cigarette substitutes.

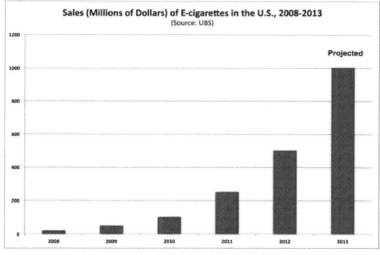

The tide is finally turning. The electronic cigarette, or e-cigarette, has emerged as the most popular of a range of smoke-free products. E-cigarettes have enjoyed explosive sales growth, doubling every year since 2008 (Figure 1). Bonnie Herzog, tobacco analyst with Wells Fargo Securities, suggests that American sales may reach $2 billion in 2013.

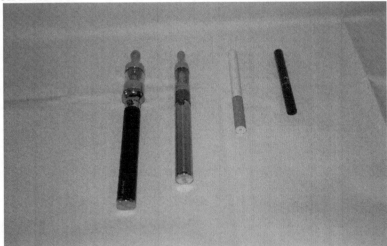

Figure 2. Variety in e-cigarettes: small single use or rechargeable models (right) and larger models producing more vapor and variable nicotine levels and flavors.

E-cigarettes are battery-powered devices that deliver a vapor of water, propylene glycol (source of the artificial smoke seen in live theaters and rock concerts), nicotine and flavorings. Users inhale the vapor through the device's mouthpiece. They're sold in a variety of styles, from small, single-use or rechargeable devices that look like cigarettes to larger models that can be modified to provide higher vapor volumes and custom nicotine levels and flavors (Figure 2). E-cigars and e-pipes are also available.

This chapter will educate you about the new kid on the harm reduction block. We'll start with a misguided – and unsuccessful – attempt by the FDA to take e-cigarettes off the market.

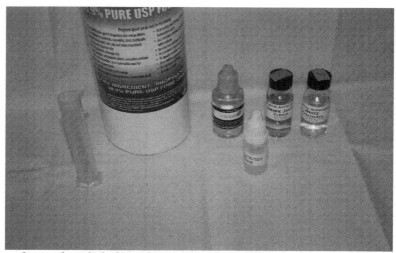

Propylene glycol (left), e-liquid (with nicotine) and flavors are used to produce customized vapor.

FDA's Attempt to Ban E-Cigarettes: "Bootstrapping Run Amuck"

E-cigarettes had been sold in the U.S. for several years when, in 2008 and 2009, the FDA detained shipments being imported by two American distributors, Smoking Everywhere and NJOY, on the grounds that the items were unapproved drug-delivery devices. The distributors filed suit in federal court and in January 2010, Judge Richard J. Leon ruled that the FDA lacked authority to regulate e-cigarettes in that manner. "The FDA," he ordered, "shall not detain or refuse admission into the United States...electronic cigarette products on the ground that those products are unapproved drugs, devices, or drug-device combinations."

The court found that the 2009 Tobacco Act "applies to 'tobacco products,' which Congress defined expansively as 'any product made or derived from tobacco that is intended for human consumption'...Congress enacted the Tobacco Act to confer FDA jurisdiction over any tobacco product – whether traditional or not –

that is sold for customary recreational use, as opposed to therapeutic use. As such, the Tobacco Act, in effect, serves as an implicit acknowledgment by Congress that FDA's jurisdiction over drugs and devices does not, and never did, extend to tobacco products, like electronic cigarettes, that are marketed in customary fashion for purely recreational purposes."

Finding that e-cigarettes, like all tobacco products, are subject to FDA oversight but fall outside of both drug and device categorization, Judge Leon characterized the FDA's attempt to apply pharmaceutical standards to e-cigarettes as "bootstrapping run amuck."

The FDA appealed and, in January 2011, lost. In an open letter published on the agency's website three months later, Center for Tobacco Products Director Dr. Lawrence R. Deyton and Center for Drug Evaluation and Research Director Dr. Janet Woodcock acknowledged that e-cigarettes are tobacco products and would be subject to regulations under the 2009 Tobacco Act. At this writing, in November 2013, no regulations have been issued.

The FDA decision was a victory on several counts for American smokers and for public health. First, the FDA guaranteed that e-cigarettes, which have helped many smokers quit, will remain on the market. Second, the Deyton-Woodcock letter indicated that the FDA will regulate e-cigarettes as to "general controls, such as registration, product listing, ingredient listing, good manufacturing practice requirements, user fees for certain products, and the adulteration and misbranding provisions, as well as to the premarket review requirements for 'new tobacco products' and 'modified risk tobacco products.'" If administered prudently, these requirements will promote the marketing of safe, quality-controlled products. Finally, the decision could allow pharmaceutical companies to reposition nicotine medicines as recreational alternatives to cigarettes.

Today, nicotine medicines are sold with a therapeutic claim for smoking cessation, but they are expensive, unsatisfying and work for only seven percent of smokers who use them. That is a dismal success rate for an FDA-approved medicine. Nothing prevents pharmaceutical companies from entering the recreational nicotine market with products that satisfy smokers indefinitely and are cheap enough to compete with cigarettes.

What's in E-Cigarette Vapor?

The vapor produced by e-cigarettes typically is made up of water, propylene glycol (PG) and nicotine. Some impurities that are present in vanishingly small amounts have been the source of persistent scaremongering.

PG is a colorless, nearly odorless, clear liquid that is commonly used in medicines, cosmetics, food, toothpaste, shampoo, mouthwash and other products. According to the FDA, PG is "generally recognized as safe" as a food additive for all food categories up to two percent.

Is PG safe? A 2011 animal study published in the journal *Toxicology* found a "relatively low toxic potential" in aerosol PG, even in high concentrations, and no impact on tissues of the voice box or lung. The researchers said the data "allowed us to conclude that [aerosol] PG exposures could be conducted safely in man by the inhalation route."

Some may object that the study only addressed the short-term health effects of inhaled PG, and no one can confidently predict that chronic exposures will be absolutely risk-free. But, it doesn't take a doctoral degree in toxicology to generally recognize that PG vapor is nowhere near as dangerous as smoke.

E-Cigarettes Effectively Deliver Nicotine

My 1995 conclusions about nicotine and cigarettes, appearing in Chapter Five, remain valid today: Nicotine is one of the most intensively studied drugs in history; while highly addictive, it is not the primary cause of *any* diseases related to smoking.

If a cigarette substitute is to be effective as a smoking-cessation, harm reduction tool, it should satisfy a smoker's craving for nicotine. E-cigarettes meet that test.

Based on research involving medicinal nicotine inhalers, e-cigarette users apparently absorb nicotine through the tissue lining their mouth and throat. A 2010 clinical trial that compared smokers' reactions to nicotine inhalers and e-cigarettes found that e-cigs produce far less mouth and throat irritation than medicinal inhalers, more "pleasant" reactions, and (for smokers) a welcome cigarette-like impact on body processes. Combined, this led the scientists to find that e-cigs have the "potential to help people stop smoking in the same way as a nicotine inhalator."

More evidence that e-cigarettes can satisfy smokers' nicotine craving was provided in a small 2013 study conducted at Virginia Commonwealth University that was published in the journal *Nicotine & Tobacco Research*. Monitoring blood nicotine levels and heart rates in smokers-turned-vapors, scientists found that e-cigs provided fast and effective nicotine satisfaction in a manner similar to cigarettes. Getting that quick hit is important to smokers; it can mean the difference between success and failure for a cigarette substitute.

Interestingly, the Virginia researchers concluded that "One important potential benefit of e-cigarette regulation may be more consistent nicotine delivery, device performance, and cartridge and vapor content." That is perfectly reasonable, but the e-cigarette community correctly fears that regulation will impose barriers to smokers' access to these life-saving products.

Should E-Cigarette Users Worry About Impurities?

In the several small e-cigarette safety studies that have been reported, no significant problems with impurities have been found.

An early study by Health New Zealand in 2008 on the liquid in Ruyan e-cigarettes (one of the original Chinese brands) found trace levels of tobacco-specific nitrosamines (TSNAs) (approximately 4 parts per billion) and some other agents. They failed to find numerous other toxic agents and heavy metals that are present in cigarette smoke. Altogether, that amounted to a rather positive safety profile.

University of California-Riverside researchers in 2013 published data showing that trace metals delivered by e-cigarettes were at levels below the daily exposure limits permitted by the authoritative U.S. Pharmacopeial Convention (USP) for inhalable medications – another positive report.

The UC-Riverside scientists cast their findings in negative terms, comparing e-cigs to cigarettes. They never made the useful comparison (above) of trace metal levels in e-cigs and USP standards. That sort of stilted reporting minimizes consumer access to the remarkably positive tobacco harm reduction potential of smoke-free tobacco products; it's a disservice to smokers and an impediment to rational pubic dialogue.

Scare Tactics

All too often, anti-tobacco zealotry trumps science. A case in point is a 2009 FDA publicity stunt that blew insignificant lab findings into an e-cigarette cancer scare. "[Our] tests indicate that these products contained detectable levels of known carcinogens" claimed the agency's press release. The feds were blowing smoke.

The agency had analyzed 18 cartridges from two e-cigarette manufacturers, gauging the levels of four tobacco-specific nitrosamines (TSNAs). Research in which I participated had earlier shown that TSNAs are present in most American tobacco products at extremely low levels, about 0.1 to 12 parts per million by weight. There is abundant scientific evidence that exposure at this level is not associated with any cancer in smokeless tobacco users. In its 2009 research, the FDA tested e-cigs using a method that detects TSNAs at about 1 million times lower concentrations than are even possibly related to human health.

In a totally unprofessional manner, the FDA chose to report only whether TSNAs were detected, rather than how much was detected. For hundreds of years, one of the basic principles of medicine has been: "The dose makes the poison." In other words, it's not the presence of a dangerous substance that we should worry about; it's the concentration, level or amount of the material present that should concern us. The FDA knew this, but chose to shout "Fire!" and hide the critical data.

This case of biased, botched research and reporting (at taxpayer expense) had yet another major wrinkle. The agency acknowledged using a Nicotrol inhaler – an FDA-approved pharmaceutical nicotine product – "as a control for some test methods," but it never actually tested that product for TSNAs. Why did the FDA analyze e-cigarettes for carcinogens, when there is no evidence the agency ever conducted carcinogen studies of products that they have approved and regulated for over 20 years?

The answer may be that the agency was trying to stifle the e-cigarette market or ban the category outright, in concert with the broader movement to prohibit all tobacco sales. Given that e-cigarettes and other smoke-free cigarette alternatives are 99 percent safer than smoking, the FDA should not disrespect science and transparency in order to justify a ban.

Another Scare Tactic: The Gateway to Nowhere

Tobacco opponents in government and elsewhere often raise a hue and cry about "THE CHILDREN!" The tactic is simple and often successful: Claim that a product or practice will lull children into bad habits and call for a ban. Earlier this year, CDC director Dr. Tom Frieden claimed in an interview with Medscape that "...many kids are starting out with e-cigarettes and then going on to smoke conventional cigarettes."

This is pure, unfounded conjecture. As of this writing, there is no scientific evidence that e-cigs are a gateway to cigarettes. Zero. Nada. None.

E-cigarette detractors are using the same gateway playbook they've used with smokeless tobacco. With not a shred of evidence, they claim that smokeless tobacco leads to smoking.

UAB epidemiologist Philip Cole and I addressed this issue in a study published in 2010. We used data from the National Survey on Drug Use and Health (NSDUH), which reveals when participants first used each tobacco product. A gateway is possible only if someone reports using smokeless tobacco (or e-cigarettes) *before* starting to smoke.

Our results did not support the hypothesis that smokeless tobacco use is a gateway to smoking at any age, including teen years. In fact, there is evidence that, compared with cigarette initiators, smokeless tobacco initiators are significantly less likely to smoke, which suggests that smokeless tobacco may actually play a protective role. The same is likely to be true for e-cigarettes.

Let me be perfectly clear: Preventing youth access to tobacco is vitally important, but this isn't a children's issue. The 8 million Americans who will die from a smoking-related illness in the next 20 years are not children. They are now adults who are at least 35 years old. It is intolerable for anti-tobacco activists to misuse a hypothetical and unproven concern about children to condemn smoking parents and grandparents to premature death.

Dual Use, Double Standard

Tobacco prohibitionists complain that some smokers will use e-cigarettes where they can't smoke, and in so doing, will remain committed smokers. There's no evidence to support this "dual-use" argument. If anything, it underscores the effectiveness of e-cigarettes as smoking substitutes.

The bogus dual-use claim has been lodged against smokeless tobacco for years. In a 2002 journal commentary, Dr. Jack Henningfield and colleagues described the theoretical adverse consequences of dual use. Despite his concerns, he acknowledged that "There are virtually no data that currently exist on the safety of such [smokeless tobacco] use or the degree to which such [smokeless tobacco] use will foster the perpetuation of smoking or contribute to reduced overall smoking."

Henningfield was wrong. Scientific evidence shows that dual smokeless tobacco users are more likely than exclusive smokers to quit smoking, but less likely to quit tobacco altogether. In one American study, 80% of exclusive smokers were still smoking at a 4-year follow-up, while only 27% of dual users were smoking. The differences between smokers and dual users in Swedish follow-up studies were even more impressive.

The bottom line: Scientific research shows that dual use is not a problem at all.

Canada Supports Marijuana Vapor, But Not Tobacco Vapor

On tobacco issues, Canada's federal health authority, Health Canada, perfectly illustrates the meaning of irrational public health policy.

The agency has blocked importation, advertising and sales of nicotine vapor systems, including e-cigarettes, since 2009, yet they support vapor delivery systems for THC (tetrahydrocannabinol), the active ingredient in marijuana.

Health Canada's website advises health professionals of "The advantages of vaporization … [of] the cannabis material" compared to the *smoking* of weed. "The subjective effects and plasma concentrations of THC are comparable to those of smoked cannabis with absorption being somewhat faster with the vaporizer. The vaporizer is well-tolerated, with no reported adverse effects, and is generally preferred over smoking by most subjects…"

On the web, Canadian health officials extensively cite a 2007 University of California at San Francisco study that emphasized the relative safety of vaping THC, rather than smoking it. "Vaporization of marijuana does not result in exposure to combustion gases, and therefore is expected to be much safer than smoking marijuana cigarettes," it reported. "The vaporizer was well tolerated and preferred by most subjects compared to marijuana cigarettes."

The study's senior author was Dr. Neal Benowitz, a former member of the FDA Tobacco Products Scientific Advisory Committee. It is perplexing that Dr. Benowitz took a rational, scientific position with respect to a "much safer" (his words) delivery system for marijuana, but has rejected the same harm reduction technology for tobacco. If vaporization is safer than combustion, why deny cigarette smokers a product that could save hundreds of thousands of lives?

The Science Says: E-Cigarettes Promote Smoking Cessation

Two 2013 clinical trials offer evidence that e-cigarettes help smokers quit or reduce cigarette consumption.

An Italian study followed 300 smokers who were *not* interested in quitting. They were split into three groups and each was given e-cigarettes with different nicotine concentrations. Data were collected at eight and 12 months. At year's end, 8.7 percent reported they had quit smoking entirely; another 10 percent reported they were smoking less. Withdrawal symptoms were seen only occasionally and weight gain was not observed at all.

These results are impressive, but they could have been better. Participants complained about the quality of the e-cigarettes they were given. "Many respondents complained of the frequent failures, lack of durability, difficulty of use (it takes time to familiarize with the puffing technique), and poor taste of the product tested." With the substantial improvements in product design and function that have been made since the trial was initiated in 2010, higher success rates might be expected if the study was redone today.

A second clinical trial reported that e-cigarettes are about as effective as nicotine patches in helping smokers quit. That should – but won't – silence critics who insist that e-cigarettes are unproven and that medicinal nicotine products are the only scientifically valid cessation aids.

The study, conducted in New Zealand, compared quit rates among 657 smokers treated for 12 weeks with nicotine e-cigarettes, nicotine-free e-cigarettes, or 21-mg. nicotine patches. There were no significant differences between any of the treatments in any time period. Six percent of smokers using nicotine patches were not smoking after six months, and seven percent of nicotine e-cigarette users had quit.

A seven-percent solution is not ideal. However, the problem may not be with e-cigarettes, but with the clinical trial model, in which smoking is the "illness," 12 weeks of e-cigarette use is the "therapy," and nicotine/tobacco abstinence is the only "outcome" acceptable to anti-tobacco activists. Most people consider smoking a lifestyle choice, not an illness; they aren't seeking treatment, and they are unwilling or unable to abstain. The real challenge is to design clinical trials to accommodate smokers' preferences and incorporate the principles of tobacco harm reduction. Changing the targeted outcome from nicotine/tobacco abstinence to smoking abstinence would permit ex-smokers to use alternative products at satisfying doses, indefinitely if they choose.

The E-Cigarette Revolution is Unstoppable

The e-cigarette revolution gained momentum when major cigarette manufacturers entered the market. In April 2012, Lorillard purchased blu e-Cigs. Three months later, RJ Reynolds launched its

VUSE e-cigarette in limited test markets. British American Tobacco announced in December 2012 that it had purchased CN Creative, maker of Intellicig e-cigarettes and Ecopure nicotine solution. BAT also owns Nicoventures, a company devoted to providing "...a new choice to smokers looking for a safer alternative to cigarettes." Altria in August 2013 launched its Mark Ten e-cigarette brand in Indiana.

Wells Fargo analyst Bonnie Herzog advised in June 2013 that "...we now anticipate the e-cig market will approach $2 billion in retail sales (including online) by the end of 2013 and eclipse $10 billion by 2017."

Herzog also noted that a steep decline in cigarette consumption would affect state payments from the 1998 Master Settlement Agreement. While cigarette manufacturers promised to pay the 46 MSA states about $206 billion over more than 20 years, their payments will be reduced if cigarette sales decline. This could lead state governments to impose excise taxes on e-cigarettes to cover those losses.

So far, e-cigarettes have not been burdened with excise taxes because they are not classified as tobacco products. The 2011 federal court ruling, however, did brand them as tobacco products. Legislators and regulators can encourage smokers to switch to healthier e-cigarettes by keeping excise taxes and burdensome regulations low or nonexistent.

The global public health implications of safer cigarette substitutes were well summarized by Sweanor *et al.* in 2007: "The relative safety of smokeless tobacco and other smoke-free systems for delivering nicotine demolishes the claim that abstinence-only approaches to tobacco are rational public health campaigns...Applying harm reduction principles to public health policies on tobacco/nicotine is more than simply a rational and humane policy. It is more than a pragmatic response to a market that is, anyway, already in the process of undergoing significant changes. It has the potential to lead to one of the greatest public health breakthroughs in human history by fundamentally changing the forecast of a billion cigarette-caused deaths this century."

he tobacco harm reduction revolution is unstoppable, and e-cigarettes are poised to play a major role.

~ ~ ~

Bibliography by Chapters

INTRODUCTION

Dole VP and Nyswander ME. A medical treatment for diacetylmorphine (heroin) addiction. *Journal of the American Medical Association* 193 (1965): 146-150.

Dole VP and Singer B. On the evaluation of treatments for narcotics addiction. *Journal of Drug Issues* 9 (1979): 205-211.

Ernster VL, Grady DG, Stillman L, Walsh M, and Greene JC. Smokeless tobacco in professional baseball: patterns of players' use. In Smokeless Tobacco or Health: An International Perspective. US Dept of Health and Human Services, Public Health Service, National Institutes of Health, NIH Publication No. 93-3461.

Glynn TJ, Boyd GM, and Gruman JC. Essential elements of self-help/minimal intervention strategies for smoking cessation. *Health Education Quarterly* 17 (1990): 329.

Hensrud DD and Sprafka JM. The smoking habits of Minnesota physicians. *American Journal of Public Health* 83 (1993): 415-417.

Nelson DE, Giovino GA, Emont SL, Brackbill R, Cameron LL, Peddicord J, and Mowery PD. Trends in cigarette smoking among United States physicians and nurses. *Journal of the American Medical Association* 271 (1994): 1273-1275.

Newman RG and Peyser N. Methadone treatment: experiment and experience. *Journal of Psychoactive Drugs* 23 (1991): 115-121.

Payte JT. A brief history of methadone in the treatment of opioid dependence: a personal perspective. *Journal of Psychoactive Drugs* 23 (1991): 103-107.

CHAPTER TWO

Axton WF. *Tobacco and Kentucky*. University Press of Kentucky, 1975.

Christen AG, Swanson BZ, Glover ED, and Henderson AH. Smokeless tobacco: the folklore and social history of snuffing, sneezing, dipping, and chewing. *Journal of the American Dental Association* 105 (1982): 821-829.

Doll R and Hill AB. Smoking and carcinoma of the lung. *British Medical Journal* 2 (1950): 739-748.

Harrison DFN. Snuff — its use and abuse. *British Medical Journal* 2 (1964); 1649-1651.

Manning WG, Keeler EB, Newhouse JP, Sloss EM, and Wasserman J. The taxes of sin: do smokers and drinkers pay their way. *Journal of the American Medical Association* 261 (1989): 1604-1609.

Sobel R. *They Satisfy: The Cigarette in American Life*. Anchor Books (Anchor Press/Doubleday). Garden City, New York, 1978.

Taylor P. *The Smoke Ring: Tobacco, Money, and Multinational Politics*. New American Library. New York, New York, 1985.

Tennant RB. *The American Cigarette Industry. A Study in Economic Analysis and Public Policy*. Yale University Press and Archon Books, 1950, 1971.

Wynder EL and Graham EA. Tobacco smoking as a possible etiologic factor in bronchogenic carcinoma. A study of six hundred and eighty-four proved cases. *Journal of the American Medical Association* 143 (1950): 329-336.

CHAPTER THREE

Allred EN, Bleecker ER, Chaitman BR, Dahms TE, et al. Short-term effects of carbon monoxide exposure on the exercise performance of subjects with coronary artery disease. *New England Journal of Medicine* 321 (1989): 1426-1432.

Bartecchi CE, MacKenzie TD, and Schrier RW. The human costs of tobacco use (Part I). *New England Journal of Medicine* 330 (1994): 907-912.

Bolinder G, Alfredsson L, Englund A, and de Faire U. Smokeless tobacco use and increased cardiovascular mortality among Swedish construction workers. *American Journal of Public Health* 84 (1994): 399-404.

Boring CC, Squires TS, Tong T. Cancer statistics 1993. *CA, A Journal for Clinicians* (American Cancer Society) 43 (1993): 7-26.

Buist AS, Ghezzo H, Anthonisen NR, et al. Relationship between the single-breath N_2 test and age, sex, and smoking habit in three North American cities. *American Review of Respiratory Diseases* 120 (1979): 305-318.

Buist AS, Sexton GJ, Nagy JM, and Ross BB. The effect of smoking cessation and modification on lung function. *American Review of Respiratory Diseases* 114 (1976): 115-122.

Carstensen JM, Pershagen G, and Eklund G. Mortality in relation to cigarette and pipe smoking: 16 years' observation of 25,000 Swedish men. *Journal of Epidemiology and Community Health* 41 (1987): 16-72.

Castelli WP. Diet, smoking, and alcohol: influence on coronary heart disease risk. *American Journal of Kidney Diseases* 16 Suppl 1 (1990): 41-46.

Centers for Disease Control and Prevention. Chronic Disease Reports: Coronary Heart Disease Mortality — United States, 1986. *Morbidity and Mortality Weekly Report* 38 (1989): 285-288.

Centers for Disease Control and Prevention. Cigarette smoking among adults — United States 1991. *Morbidity and Mortality Weekly Report* 42 (1993): 230-233.

Centers for Disease Control and Prevention. Cigarette smoking-attributable mortality and years of potential life lost — United States, 1990. *Morbidity and Mortality Weekly Report* 42 (1993): 645-649.

Centers for Disease Control and Prevention. State-specific estimates of smoking-attributable mortality and years of potential life lost — United States, 1985. *Morbidity and Mortality Weekly Report* 37 (1988): 689-694.

Chang HH, Lininger LL, Doyle JT, Maccubbin PA, and Rothenberg RB. Application of the Cox model as a predictor of relative risk of coronary heart disease in the Albany study. *Statistics in Medicine* 9 (1990): 287-292.

Goldman L and Cook F. The decline in ischemic heart disease mortality rates. An analysis of the comparative effects of medical interventions and changes in lifestyle. *Annals of Internal Medicine* 101 (1984): 825-836.

Higgins M and Thom T. Trends in coronary heart disease in the United States. *International Journal of Epidemiology* 18 (1989): S58-S66.

Huhtasaari F, Asplund K, Lundberg V, Stegmayr B, and Wester PO. Tobacco and myocardial infarction: is snuff less dangerous than cigarettes? *British Medical Journal* 305 (1992): 1252-1256.

Kaufman DW, Helmrich SP, Rosenberg L, Miettinen OS, and Shapiro S. Nicotine and carbon monoxide content of cigarette smoke and the risk of myocardial infarction in young men. *New England Journal of Medicine* 308 (1983): 409-413.

LaCroix AZ, Lang J, Scherr P, et al. Smoking and mortality among older men and women in three communities. *New England Journal of Medicine* 324 (1991): 1619-1625.

MacKenzie TD, Bartecchi CE, and Schrier RW. The human costs of tobacco use (Part II). *New England Journal of Medicine* 330 (1994): 975-980.

Mera SL, Atherosclerosis and coronary heart disease. *British Journal of the Biomedical Sciences* 50 (1993): 235-248.

Rice DP, Hodgson TA, Sinsheimer P, Browner W, and Kopstein AN. The economic costs of the health effects of smoking, 1984. The Milbank Quarterly 64 (1986): 489-547. The Milbank Memorial Fund.

Rosenberg L, Kaufman DW, Helmrich SP, and Shapiro S. The risk of myocardial infarction after quitting smoking in men under 55 years of age. *New England Journal of Medicine* 313 (1985): 1511-1514.

Rosenberg L, Palmer JR, and Shapiro S. Decline of the risk of myocardial infarction among women who stop smoking. *New England Journal of Medicine* 322 (1990): 213-217.

Samet JM, Wiggins CL, Humble CG, and Pathak DR. Cigarette smoking and lung cancer in New Mexico. *American Review of Respiratory Diseases* 137 (1988): 1110-1113.

Sleight P. Cardiovascular risk factors and the effects of intervention. *American Heart Journal* 121 (1991): 990-995.

Subar AF and Harlan LC. Nutrient and food group intake by tobacco use status: the 1987 national health interview survey. *Annals of the New York Academy of Sciences* 686 (1993): 310-321.

US Department of Health and Human Services: Reducing the health consequences of smoking: 25 years of progress. A Report of the Surgeon General. US Department of Health and Human Services, Public Health Service, Centers for Disease Control, Center for Chronic Disease Prevention and Health Promotion, Office on Smoking and Health. DHHS Publication No (CDC) 89-8411, 1989.

US Department of Health and Human Services: The health benefits of smoking cessation. A Report of the Surgeon General. US Department of Health and Human Services, Public Health Service, Office of the Assistant Secretary for Health, Office on Smoking and Health. DHHS Publication No (CDC) 90-8416, 1990.

US Department of Health and Human Services: The health consequences of smoking: cardiovascular disease. A Report of the Surgeon General. US Department of Health and Human Services, Public Health Service, Office of the Assistant Secretary for Health, Office on Smoking and Health. DHHS Publication No (PHS) 84-50204, 1983.

Wolf PA, D'Agostino RB, Kannel WB, Bonita R, and Belanger AJ. Cigarette smoking as a risk factor for stroke. The Framingham Study. *Journal of the American Medical Association* 259 (1988): 1025-1030.

CHAPTER FOUR

Blot WJ and Fraumeni JF. Passive smoking and lung cancer. *Journal of the National Cancer Institute* 77 (1986): 993-1000.

Boyle P. The hazards of passive — and active — smoking. *New England Journal of Medicine* 328 (1993): 1708-1709.

Byrd JC. Environmental tobacco smoke: medical and legal issues. *Medical Clinics of North America* 76 (1992): 377-398.

Chilmonczyk BA, Salmun LM, Megathlin KN, Neveux LM, Palomaki GE, Knight GJ, Pulkkinen AJ, and Haddow JE. Association between exposure to environmental tobacco smoke and exacerbations of asthma in children. *New England Journal of Medicine* 328 (1993): 1665-1669.

Fielding JE and Phenow KJ. Health effects of involuntary smoking. *New England Journal of Medicine* 319 (1988): 1452-1460.

Fontham ETH, Correa P, Reynolds P, Wu-Williams A, Buffler PA, Greenberg RS, et al. Environmental tobacco smoke and lung cancer in nonsmoking women: a multicenter study. *Journal of the American Medical Association* 271 (1994): 1752-1759.

Gallup G Jr. and Newport F. Many Americans favor restrictions on smoking in public places. *Gallup Poll Monthly* 298 (1990): 19.

Gori GB. Science, policy, and ethics: the case of environmental tobacco smoke. *Journal of Clinical Epidemiology* 47 (1994): 325-334.

Luik JC. Pandora's box: the dangers of politically corrupted science for democratic public policy. *Bostonian*, Winter (1993-94): pp 50-60.

Martinez FD, Cline M, and Burrows B. Increased incidence of asthma in children of smoking mothers. *Pediatrics* 89 (1992): 21-26.

Miller AL. The United States smoking-material fire problem through 1990: the role of lighted tobacco products in fire. Quincy, MA: National Fire Protection Association, 1993.

Office of Health and Environmental Assessment, Office of Research and Development. Respiratory Health Effects of Passive Smoking: Lung Cancer and Other Disorders. Washington, D.C.: United States Environmental Protection Agency, 1992.

Taylor AE, Johnson DC, and Kazemi H. Environmental tobacco smoke and cardiovascular disease. A position paper from the Council on Cardiopulmonary and Critical Care, American Heart Association. *Circulation* 86 (1992): 699-702.

Weiss ST. Passive smoking and lung cancer: what is the risk? *American Review of Respiratory Diseases* 133 (1986): 1-3.

Weitzman M, Gortmaker S, Walker DK, and Sobol A. Maternal smoking and childhood asthma. *Pediatrics* 85 (1990): 505-511.

CHAPTER FIVE

Benowitz, NL. Pharmacologic aspects of cigarette smoking and nicotine addiction. *New England Journal of Medicine* 319 (1988): 1318-1330.

Bittoun R. Recurrent aphthous ulcers and nicotine. *Medical Journal of Australia* 154 (1991): 471-472.

Fagerström KO, Schneider NG. Measuring nicotine dependence: a review of the Fagerström Tolerance Questionnaire. *Journal of Behavioral Medicine* 12 (1989): 159-182.

Hanauer SB. Nicotine for colitis — the smoke has not yet cleared. *New England Journal of Medicine* 330 (1994): 856-857.

Hughes JR, Higgins ST, Hatsukami D. Effects of abstinence from tobacco. A critical review. In Kozlowski LT, Annis HM, Cappell HD, et al (eds). Research Advances in Alcohol and Drug Problems. New York, Plenum Publishing Corporation, 1990.

Jarvik ME. Beneficial effects of nicotine. *British Journal of Addiction* 86 (1992): 571-575.

Johnston LM. Tobacco smoking and nicotine. *The Lancet* 243 (2) (1942): 742.

King A. *The Cigarette Habit: A Scientific Cure*. Doubleday and Co., Inc. Garden City, New York. 1959.

Koskowski W. *The Habit of Tobacco Smoking*. Staples Press Limited, London. 1955.

Kozlowski LT, Wilkinson A, Skinner W, Kent C, Franklin T, and Pope M. Comparing tobacco dependence with other drug dependencies. *Journal of the American Medical Association* 261 (1989): 898-901.

Larson PS, Haag HB, and Silvette H. *Tobacco: Experimental and Clinical Studies*. A Comprehensive Account of the World Literature. Williams and Wilkins Co., Baltimore, 1961.

Lashner BA, Hanauer SB, and Silverstein MD. Testing nicotine gum for ulcerative colitis patients: experience with single-patient trials. *Digestive Disease and Science* 35 (1990): 827-832.

London ED, Waller SB, and Wamsley JK. Autographic localization of ^{3}H nicotine binding sites in rat brains. *Neurosciences Letter* 53 (1985): 179-184.

Martin WR, Van Loon GR, Iwamoto ET, and Davis LD. *Tobacco Smoking and Nicotine: A Neurobiological Approach*. Plenum Press, New York, 1987.

Ockrene JK (ed). The Pharmacologic Treatment of Tobacco Dependence: Proceedings of the World Congress, November 4-5, 1985. Cambridge, MA: Institute for the Study of Smoking Behavior and Policy, 1986.

Pomerleau OF and Pomerleau CS. Neuroregulators and the reinforcement of smoking: towards a biobehavioral explanation. *Neurosciences and Biobehavioral Reviews* 8 (1984): 503-513.

Pullan RD, Rhodes J, Ganesh S, Mani V, Morris JS, Williams GT et al. Transdermal nicotine for active ulcerative colitis. *New England Journal of Medicine* 330 (1994): 811-815.

Russell MAH, Jarvis MJ, West RJ, and Feyerabend C. Buccal absorption of nicotine from smokeless tobacco sachets. *The Lancet* 8468 (1985): 1370.

Sahakian B, Jones G, Levy R, Gray J, and Warburton D. Effects of nicotine on attention, information processing, and short-term memory in patients with dementia of the Alzheimer type. *British Journal of Psychiatry* 154 (1989): 797-800.

US Department of Health and Human Services: The health consequences of smoking: nicotine addiction. A Report of the Surgeon General. US Department of Health and Human Services, Public Health Service, Centers for Disease Control, Center for Chronic Disease Prevention and Health Promotion, Office on Smoking and Health. DHHS Publication No. (PHS) 88-8406, 1988.

CHAPTER SIX

Baile WF Jr., Bigelow GE, Gottlieb SH, Stitzer ML, and Sacktor JD. Rapid resumption of cigarette smoking following myocardial infarction: inverse relation to MI severity. *Addictive Behaviors* 7 (1982): 373-380.

Benowitz NL, Jacob P III and Savanapridi C. Determinants of nicotine intake while chewing nicotine polacrilex gum. *Clinical Pharmacology and Therapeutics* 41 (1987): 467-473.

Benowitz NL. Pharmacologic aspects of cigarette smoking and nicotine addiction. *New England Journal of Medicine* 319 (1988): 1318-1330.

Ejrup B and Wikander PA. Fortsatta forsoktill avvanjing fran tobak medelst injektions behandling. *Svenska Lakartidn* 56 (1959): 1975.

Emont SL and Cummings KM. Weight gain following smoking cessation: a possible role for nicotine replacement in weight management. *Addictive Behaviors* 12 (1987): 151-155.

Fagerström KO. Reducing the weight gain after stopping smoking. *Addictive Behaviors* 12 (1987): 91-93.

Fisher EB, Haire-Joshu D, Morgan GD, Rehberg H, and Rost K. Smoking and smoking cessation. *American Review of Respiratory Diseases* 142 (1990): 702-706.

Fisher EB, Lichtenstein E, Haire-Joshu D, Morgan GD, and Rehberg HR. Methods, successes, and failures of smoking cessation programs. *Annual Review of Medicine* 44 (1993): 481-513.

Fiore MC, Jorenby DE, Baker TB, and Kenford SL. Tobacco dependence and the nicotine patch: clinical guides for effective use. *Journal of the American Medical Association* 268 (1992): 2687-2694.

Fiore MC, Novotny TE, Pierce JP, et al. Methods used to quit smoking in the United States: Do cessation programs help? *Journal of the American Medical Association* 263 (1990): 2760-2765.

Gross J, Stitzer ML, and Maldonado J. Nicotine replacement: effects on postcessation weight gain. *Journal of Consulting and Clinical Psychology* 57 (1989): 87-92.

Hajek P, Jackson P, and Belcher M. Long-term use of nicotine chewing gum: occurrence, determinants, and effect on weight gain. *Journal of the American Medical Association* 260 (1988): 1593-1598.

Hatziandreu EJ, Pierce JP, Lefkopoulou M, et al. Quitting smoking in the United States. *Journal of the National Cancer Institute* 82 (1990): 1402-1406.

Hughes JR. Problems of nicotine gum. In Ockene, JK (ed). The Pharmacologic Treatment of Tobacco Dependence: Proceedings of the World Conference. Cambridge, MA, Institute for the Study of Smoking Behavior and Policy 141, 1986.

Lam W, Sze PC, Sacks HS, and Chalmers TC. Meta-analysis of randomised controlled trials of nicotine chewing-gum. *The Lancet* 2 (1987): 27-30.

McNabb ME. Chewing nicotine gum for 3 months: what happens to plasma nicotine levels? *Canadian Medical Association Journal* 131 (1984): 589-592.

Norregaard J, Tonnesen P, Simonsen K, and Sawe U. Long-term nicotine substitution after application of a 16-hour nicotine patch in smoking cessation. *European Journal of Pharmacology* 43 (1992): 57-60.

Schneider NG. Nicotine therapy in smoking cessation: pharmacokinetic considerations. *Clinical Pharmacokinetics* 23 (1992): 169-172.

Schwartz JL. Methods of smoking cessation. *Medical Clinics of North America* 76 (1992): 451-476.

Schwid SS, Hirvonen MD, and Keesey RE. Nicotine effects on body weight: a regulatory perspective. *American Journal of Clinical Nutrition* 55 (1992): 878-884.

Silagy C, Mant D, Fowler G, and Lodge M. Meta-analysis on efficacy of nicotine replacement therapies in smoking cessation. *The Lancet* 343 (1994): 139-142.

Tonnesen P, Norregaard J, Simonsen K, Sawe U. A double-blind trial of a 16-hour transdermal nicotine patch in smoking cessation. *New England Journal of Medicine* 325 (1991): 311-315.

CHAPTER SEVEN

American Cancer Society. Smokeless tobacco could cause national epidemic. *Cancer News* 47 (1993): 22.

Axell T, Mornstad H, and Sundstrom B. The relation of the clinical picture to the histopathology of snuff dipper's lesions in a Swedish population. *Journal of Oral Pathology* 5 (1976): 229-236.

Benowitz NL. Pharmacologic aspects of cigarette smoking and nicotine addiction. *New England Journal of Medicine* 319 (1988): 1318-1330.

Blot WJ, McLaughlin JK, Winn DM, et al. Smoking and drinking in relation to oral and pharyngeal cancer. *Cancer Research* 48 (1988): 3282-3287.

Boring, CC, Squires, TS, Tong, T. Cancer statistics 1993. *CA, A Journal for Clinicians* (American Cancer Society) 43 (1993): 7-26.

Bouquot J, Schroeder K. Oral leukoplakia and smokeless tobacco keratoses are two separate and distinctive precancers. *Oral Surgery, Oral Medicine, Oral Pathology* 76 (1993): 588-589.

CA, A Journal for Clinicians (American Cancer Society), Cancer Statistics, 1960-1983.

Centers for Disease Control and Prevention. Use of smokeless tobacco among adults — United States, 1991. *Morbidity and Mortality Weekly Report* 42 (1993); 263-265.

Christen, AG, Swanson, BZ, Glover, ED, and Henderson, AH. Smokeless tobacco: the folklore and social history of snuffing, sneezing, dipping, and chewing. *Journal of the American Dental Association* 105 (1982): 821-829.

Cullen JW, Blot W, Henningfield J, Boyle G, Mecklenburg R, Massey MM. Health consequences of using smokeless tobacco: summary of the advisory committee's report to the surgeon general. *Public Health Reports* 101 (1986): 355-373.

Grady D, Greene J, Daniels TE et al. Oral mucosal lesions found in smokeless tobacco users. *Journal of the American Dental Association* 121 (1990): 117-123.

Greene JC, Ernster VL, Grady DG, Robertson PB, Walsh MM and Stillman LA. Oral mucosal lesions: Clinical findings in relation to smokeless tobacco use among United States baseball players. *Monograph. 2; Smokeless Tobacco or Health, An International Perspective* 41-50. NIH publication No 93-3461.

Hatsukami D, Nelson R, and Jensen J. Smokeless tobacco: current status and future directions. *British Journal of Addiction* 86 (1991): 559-563.

Huhtasaari F, Asplund K, Lundberg V, Stegmayr B, and Wester PO. Tobacco and myocardial infarction: is snuff less dangerous than cigarettes. *British Medical Journal* 305 (1992): 1252-1256.

Mason TJ and McKay FW. United States Cancer Mortality by County: 1950-1969. US Department of Health and Human Services, Public Health Service, National Institutes of Health, National Cancer Institute, DHEW Publication No (NIH) 74-615, 1974.

Nordgren P, Ramström L. Moist snuff in Sweden — tradition and evolution. *British Journal of Addiction* 85 (1990): 1107-1112.

Palmer C. Dr. Novello targets smokeless. *American Dental Association News*, January 4, 1993.

Riggan WB, Van Bruggen J, Acquavella JF, Beaubier J, and Mason TJ. United States Cancer Mortality Rates and Trends, 1950-1979, Volume I. National Cancer Institute and United States Environmental Protection Agency. NCI/EPA Interagency Agreement on Environmental Carcinogenesis, 1983.

Rodu B. An alternative approach to smoking control. *American Journal of the Medical Sciences* 308 (1994): 32-34.

Rodu B and Cole P. Tobacco-related mortality. *Nature* 370 (1994): 184.

Rodu B and Cole P. Excess mortality in smokeless tobacco users not meaningful. *American Journal of Public Health* 85 (1995): 118.

Roed-Petersen B and Pindborg JJ. A study of snuff induced oral leukoplakias. *Journal of Oral Pathology* 2 (1973): 301-313.

Russell MAH, Jarvis MJ, West RJ and Feyerabend C. Buccal absorption of nicotine from smokeless tobacco sachets. *The Lancet* 8468 (1985): 1370.

Russell MAH, Jarvis MJ, and Feyerabend C. A new age for snuff? *The Lancet* 1 (1980): 474-475.

Sinusas K, Coroso JG, Sopher MD, and Carbtree BF. Smokeless tobacco use and oral pathology in a professional baseball organization. *Journal of Family Practice* 34 (1992): 713-718.

Smith JF, Mincer HA, Hopkins KP, and Bell J. Snuff-dipper's lesion. A cytological and pathological study in a large population. *Archives of Otolaryngology* 92 (1970): 450-456.

Smith JF. Snuff-dippers lesions. A ten-year follow-up. *Archives of Otolaryngology* 101 (1975): 276-277.

Stockwell HG and Lyman GH. Impact of smoking and smokeless tobacco on the risk of cancer of the head and neck. *Head and Neck Surgery* 9 (1986): 104-110.

Tilashalski K, Lozano K and Rodu B. Modified tobacco use as a risk-reduction strategy. *Journal of Psychoactive Drugs* 27 (1995): 173-175.

Tilashalski K, Rodu B, and Mayfield C. Assessing the nicotine content of smokeless tobacco products. *Journal of the American Dental Association* 125 (1994): 590-594.

Vigneswaran N, Tilashalski K, Rodu B and Cole P. Tobacco use and cancer: a reappraisal. *Oral Surgery, Oral Medicine, Oral Pathology* 80 (1995): 178-182.

Winn DM, Blot WJ, Shy CM, Pickle LW, Toledo A and Fraumeni JF. Snuff dipping and oral cancer among women in the southern United States. *New England Journal of Medicine* 304 (1981): 745-749.

CHAPTER EIGHT

Baker R. The Danger Stage. *New York Times*, May 31, 1994.

Benowitz NL, Henningfield JE. Establishing a nicotine threshold for addiction: the implications for tobacco regulation. *New England Journal of Medicine* 331 (1994): 123-125.

Connolly GN. Banning oral snuff. *The Lancet* 337 (1991): 1484.

Connolly GN. Worldwide expansion of transnational tobacco industry. *Journal of the National Cancer Institute Monographs* 12 (1992): 29-35.

Daynard RA. Tobacco litigation — purpose, performance, and prospects. *Journal of the National Cancer Institute Monographs* 12 (1992): 53-56.

Doron G. *The Smoking Paradox: Public Regulation in the Cigarette Industry*. Abt Books, Cambridge, MA, 1979.

Goodin RE. *No Smoking: The Ethical Issues*. The University of Chicago Press. Chicago and London, 1989.

Gray N. Evidence and overview of global tobacco problem. *Journal of the National Cancer Institute Monographs* 12 (1992): 15-16.

MacKenzie TD, Bartecchi CE, and Schrier RW. The human costs of tobacco use (Part II). *New England Journal of Medicine* 330 (1994): 975-980.

Mahar M. Tobacco's smoking gun. *Barron's*, May 16, 1994, pp 33-37.

Parry R. *Fooling America: How Washington Insiders Twist the Truth and Manufacture the Conventional Wisdom*. William Morrow and Company, Inc. New York, 1992.

Peto R, Lopez AD, Boreham J, Thun M, and Heath C, Jr. Mortality from tobacco in developed countries: indirect estimation from national vital statistics. *The Lancet* 339 (1992): 1268-1278.

Pierce JP, Thurmond L, and Rosbrook B. Projecting international lung cancer mortality rates: first approximations with tobacco-consumption data. *Journal of the National Cancer Institute Monographs* 12 (1992): 45-49.

Prevention Magazine 42 (1990): 27-28, November.

Schwartz JL. Methods of smoking cessation. *Medical Clinics of North America* 76 (1992): 451-477.

Tollison RD and Wagner RE. *The Economics of Smoking.* Kluwer Academic Publishers, Boston, MA, 1992.

Troyer RJ and Markle GE. *Cigarettes: The Battle Over Smoking.* Rutgers University Press, New Brunswick, NJ, 1983.

Tufte, ER. Improving data analysis in political science. In ER Tufte (ed): *The Quantitative Analysis of Social Science,* Addison-Wesley, Reading, MA, 1970.

US Department of Commerce National Trade Data Bank, Economic and Statistics Administration, December 1993.

The Washington Post, Health tabloid, October 19, 1993.

White LC. *Merchants of Death: The American Tobacco Industry.* Beech Tree Books (William Morrow), New York, New York, 1988.

Whelan EM. *A Smoking Gun: How the Tobacco Industry Gets Away with Murder.* George F. Stockley Co., Philadelphia, PA, 1984.

Viscusi WK. *Smoking: Making the Risky Decision.* Oxford University Press, New York and Oxford, 1992.

CHAPTER NINE

Abrams DI, Vizoso HP, Shade SB, Jay C, Kelly ME, and Benowitz NL. Vaporization as a smokeless cannabis delivery system: a pilot study. *Clinical Pharmacology and Therapeutics* 82 (2007): 572-578.

Bergström M, Nordberg A, Lunell E, Antoni G, and Långström B. Regional deposition of inhaled 11C-nicotine vapor in the human airway as visualized by positron emission tomography. *Clinical Pharmacology and Therapeutics* 57(1995): 309-317.

Bullen C, McRobbie H, Thornley S, Glover M, Lin R, and Laugesen M. Effect of an electronic nicotine delivery device (e cigarette) on desire to smoke and withdrawal, user preferences and nicotine delivery: randomized cross-over trial. *Tobacco Control* 19 (2010): 98-103.

Deyton LR, Woodcock J. Regulation of e-cigarettes and other tobacco products. U.S. Federal Drug Administration, April 25, 2011. Available   at: http://www.fda.gov/NewsEvents/PublicHealthFocus/ucm252360.htm

Eissenberg T. Electronic nicotine delivery devices: ineffective nicotine delivery and craving suppression after acute administration (letter). *Tobacco Control* 19 (2010): 87-88.

Fiore M. CDC Director on Antibiotics, Influenza, and E-Cigarettes. Medscape, September 26, 2013. Available at: http://www.medscape.com/viewarticle/811616

Frost-Pineda K, Appleton S, Fisher M, and Gaworski CL. Does dual use jeopardize the potential role of smokeless tobacco in harm reduction? *Nicotine & Tobacco Research* 12 (2010): 1055-1067.

Health Canada website. Vapourized Cannabis. Available at: http://www.hc-sc.gc.ca/dhp-mps/marihuana/med/infoprof-eng.php#chp2212

Henningfield JE, Rose CA, and Giovino GA. Brave new world of tobacco disease prevention: promoting dual tobacco-product use? *American Journal of Preventive Medicine* 23 (2002): 226-228.

Kozlowski LT, O'Connor, Edwards BQ, and Flaherty BP. Most smokeless tobacco use is not a causal gateway to cigarettes: using order of product use to evaluate causation in a national U.S. sample. *Addiction* 98 (2003): 1077-1085.

Laugesen M. Safety Report on the Ruyan® e-cigarette Cartridge and Inhaled Aerosol. Health New Zealand, 30 October 2008. Available at: http://www.healthnz.co.nz/RuyanCartridgeReport30-Oct-08.pdf

Laugesen M. Snuffing out cigarette sales and the smoking deaths epidemic. *New Zealand Medical Journal* 120 (2007): U2587.

Lunell E, Molander L, Leischow SJ, and Fagerström K.O. Effect of nicotine vapour inhalation on the relief of tobacco withdrawal symptoms. *European Journal of Clinical Pharmacology* 48 (1995): 235-240.

Mishori R: E-cigarettes: can they help you quit? Parade Magazine, July 12, 2009. Available at: http://www.parade.com/health/2009/07/12-e-cigarettes-healthy-or-not.html

O'Connor RJ, Flaherty BP, Edwards BQ, and Kozlowski LT. Regular smokeless tobacco use is not a reliable predictor of smoking onset when psychosocial predictors are included in the model. *Nicotine & Tobacco Research* 5 (2003): 535-543.

O'Connor RJ, Kozlowski LT, Flaherty BP, and Edwards BQ. Most smokeless tobacco use does not cause cigarette smoking: results from the 2000 National Household Survey on Drug Abuse. *Addictive Behaviors* 30 (2005): 325-336.

Rodu B. Dual use (letter). *Nicotine & Tobacco Research* 2011. doi: 10.1093/ntr/ntq23

Rodu B and Cole P: Nicotine maintenance for inveterate smokers. *Technology* 6 (1999): 17-21.

Rodu B and Cole P. Evidence against a gateway from smokeless tobacco use to smoking. *Nicotine & Tobacco Research* 12 (2010): 530-534.

Rodu B and Godshall WT. Tobacco harm reduction: an alternative cessation strategy for inveterate smokers. *Harm Reduction Journal* 3 (2006):37, (Open Access, available at www.harmreductionjournal.com/content/pdf/1477-7517-3-37.pdf).

Rodu B and Jansson C. Smokeless Tobacco and Oral Cancer: A Review of the Risks and Determinants. *Critical Reviews in Oral Biology and Medicine* 15 (2004); 252-263.

Rodu B, Stegmayr B, Nasic S, Cole P and Asplund K. Evolving patterns of tobacco use in northern Sweden. *Journal of Internal Medicine* 253 (2003): 660–665.

Rose JE, Turner JE, Murugesan T, Behm FM and Laugesen M. Pulmonary delivery of nicotine pyruvate: sensory and pharmacokinetic characteristics. *Experimental and Clinical Psychopharmacology* 18 (2010):385-394.

Royal College of Physicians. Harm reduction in nicotine addiction: helping people who can't quit. A report by the Tobacco Advisory Group of the Royal College of Physicians. 2007, London, United Kingdom. Available at: http://bookshop.rcplondon.ac.uk/details.aspx?e=234

Russell MAH. Realistic goals for smoking and health: a case for safer smoking. *Lancet* 1 (1974): 254-258.

Sweanor D, Alcabes P and Drucker E. Tobacco harm reduction: how rational public policy could transform a pandemic. *International Journal of Drug Policy* 18 (2007): 70-74.

Timberlake DS, Huh J and Lakon CM. Use of propensity score matching in evaluating smokeless tobacco as a gateway to smoking. *Nicotine & Tobacco Research* 11 (2009): 455-462.

Trtchounian A, Williams M and Talbot P. Conventional and electronic cigarettes (e-cigarettes) have different smoking characteristics. *Nicotine & Tobacco Research* 2010. doi: 10.1093/ntr/ntq114

U.S. Department of Health and Human Services, Food and Drug Administration, Center for Drug Evaluation and Research. Evaluation of e-cigarettes. Available at: http://www.fda.gov/downloads/Drugs/ScienceResearch/UCM17325 0.pdf

United States District Court For the District of Columbia. Civil Case No. 09-771. Memorandum Opinion by Richard. J. Leon, January 14, 2010. Available at: https://ecf.dcd.uscourts.gov/cgi-bin/show_public_doc?2009cv0771-54

Vansickel AR, Cobb CO, Weaver MF and Eissenberg TE. A clinical laboratory model for evaluating the acute effects of electronic "cigarettes": nicotine delivery profile and cardiovascular and subjective effects. *Cancer Epidemiology, Biomarkers and Prevention* 19 (2010): 1945-1953.

Vansickel AR and Eissenberg T. Electronic cigarettes: effective nicotine delivery after acute administration. *Nicotine & Tobacco Research* 15 (2013): 267-270.

Werley MS, McDonald P, Lilly P, Kirkpatrick D, Wallery J, Byron P and Venitz J. Non-clinical safety and pharmacokinetic evaluations of propylene glycol aerosol in Sprague-Dawley rats and Beagle dogs. *Toxicology* 287 (2011): 76-90.

Westenberger BJ. Deputy Director. Evaluation of e-cigarettes. Division of Pharmaceutical Analysis, U.S. Food and Drug Administration. Available at http://www.fda.gov/downloads/Drugs/ScienceResearch/UCM17325 0.pdf

Wetter DW, McClure JB, de Moor C, Cofta-Gunn L, Cummings S, Cinciripini PM and Gritz ER. Concomitant use of cigarettes and smokeless tobacco: prevalence, correlates, and predictors of tobacco cessation. *Preventive Medicine* 34 (2002): 638-648.

Williams M, Villarreal A, Bozhilov K, Lin S and Talbot P. Metal and silicate particles including nanoparticles are present in electronic cigarette cartomizer fluid and aerosol. *PLoS One* 2013, available at http://www.plosone.org/article/info%3Adoi%2F10.1371%2Fjournal.pone.0057987

~ ~ ~

BE SURE TO LISTEN TO THE "FOR SMOKERS ONLY" AUDIOBOOK AVAILABLE ON AUDIBLE.COM AND ITUNES. GO TO WWW.SUMNERBOOKS.COM.